Fitness That Works

SIMPLE MOVES TO MAKE EXERCISE HAPPEN FROM 9 TO 5

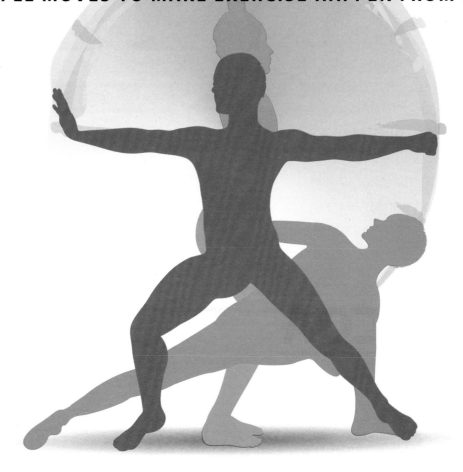

About

WELCOA

The Wellness Council of America (WELCOA) was established as a national not-for-profit organization in the mid 1980s through the efforts of a number of forward-thinking business and health leaders. Drawing on the vision originally set forth by William Kizer, Sr., Chairman Emeritus of Central States Indemnity, and WELCOA founding Directors that included Dr. Louis Sullivan, former Secretary of Health and Human Services, and Warren Buffet, Chairman of Berkshire Hathaway, WELCOA has helped influence the face of workplace wellness in the U.S.

Today, WELCOA has become one of the most respected resources for workplace wellness in America. With a membership in excess of 5,000 organizations, WELCOA is dedicated to improving the health and well-being of all working Americans. Located in America's heartland, WELCOA makes its national headquarters in one of America's healthiest business communities— Omaha, Nebraska.

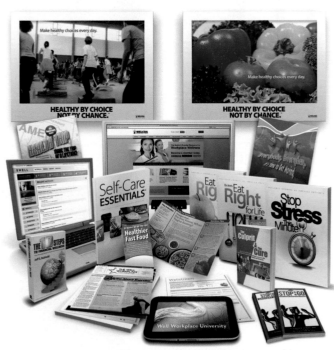

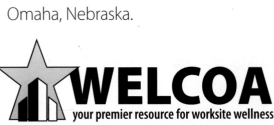

WELCOA
your premier resource for worksite wellness

17002 Marcy Street, Suite 140 | Omaha, NE 68118
PH: 402-827-3590 | FX: 402-827-3594 | welcoa.org

Editorial Staff

Author:	Sean Foy, MA
Executive Editor:	David Hunnicutt, PhD
Managing Editor:	Brittanie Leffelman, MS
Contributing Editors:	Madeline Jahn, MOL
	Carie Maguire
Multimedia Designer:	Adam Paige
Graphic Designer:	Brittany Stohl

Table Of
Contents

About...

Sean Foy, MA

Sean Foy is an internationally renowned authority on fitness, weight management and healthy living. As an author, exercise physiologist, behavioral coach and speaker, Sean has earned the reputation as "America's Fast Fitness Expert." With an upbeat, positive and sensible approach to making fitness happen even with the busiest of schedules, he has taken his message of "simple moves" fitness all over the world.

He is the author of the *10 Minute Total Body Breakthrough* and the co-creator of an award winning children's health and fitness program, LEAN KIDS. Sean is also the author and developer of the signature fitness program for *The Biggest Loser® Pro Training* program. Among numerous other awards, he received the "Nike Go" Top National Health Education Program Award and the California Governor Health Educator of the Year Award.

As a husband and father of two, as well as President and founder of Personal Wellness Corporation, an international wellness education, speaking and consulting firm, Sean understands "busy" and brings his real life exercise solutions to audiences wherever he goes. Appearing on ABC, NBC, CBN and other popular national television outlets, he has spent the last 20 years testing, researching and sharing his findings on how to crack the code to make fitness work.

Sean has helped thousands of individuals with their wellness needs as a personal trainer, counselor, presenter and business owner and is committed to encouraging everyone to attain optimal well-being for body, mind and spirit!

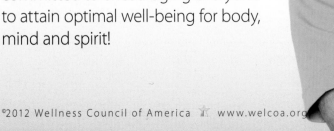

Foreword

Plain and simple, exercise is medicine. In fact, if exercise came in pill form it would be the most powerful and effective medicine the world has ever known. Still, despite its effectiveness, exercise remains elusive for many working Americans. That's why I've asked Sean Foy, one of the nation's leading experts on exercise and health, to write this book.

Soon you'll see that *Fitness That Works: Simple Moves To Make Exercise Happen From 9 To 5*, is unlike other fitness manuals. Indeed, what's unique about this book is that it provides guidance for working men and women and actually gets them up and moving at work—something that's essential to preserving human health. And by engaging everyone, this book has the power to change lives and transform organizational culture.

By leveraging simple moves that have HUGE payoff, this book will impact you and your organization in important ways. Not only will you become healthier, you'll also become happier, more productive and more engaged. And thanks to Sean Foy and his unique insights, the formula for becoming more fit is a simple one.

In closing, I'd like to thank Sean Foy for his contributions, insights, passion, and enthusiasm—there are few people as well-equipped to address this topic as Sean. And in just a few pages you'll see firsthand the power of Sean's simple and fun fitness moves.

Best of luck to you on your journey to master *Fitness That Works: Simple Moves To Make Exercise Happen From 9 To 5*.

Warmest Regards,

David Hunnicutt, PhD
President
Wellness Council of America

ABOUT DR. DAVID HUNNICUTT

Since his arrival at WELCOA in 1995, David Hunnicutt, PhD has developed countless publications that have been widely adopted in businesses and organizations throughout North America. Known for his ability to make complex issues easier to understand, David has a proven track-record of publishing health and wellness material that helps employees lead healthier lifestyles. David travels extensively advocating better health practices and radically different thinking in organizations of all kinds

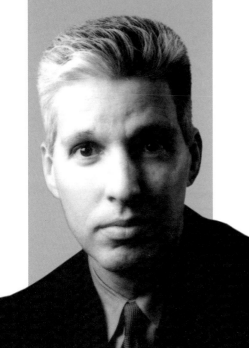

Introduction...
Get Movin'

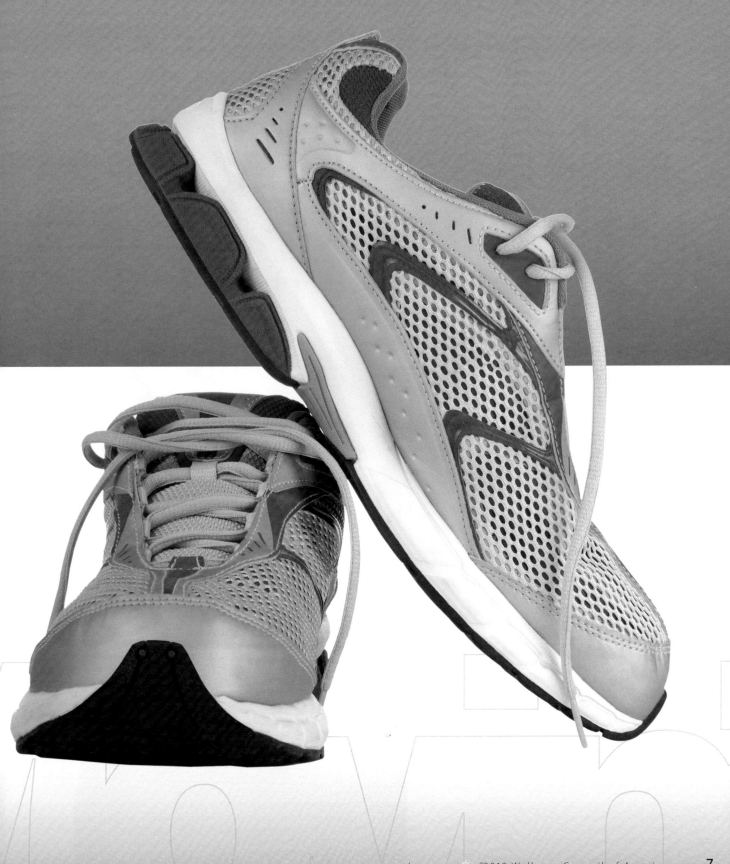

Get Movin'

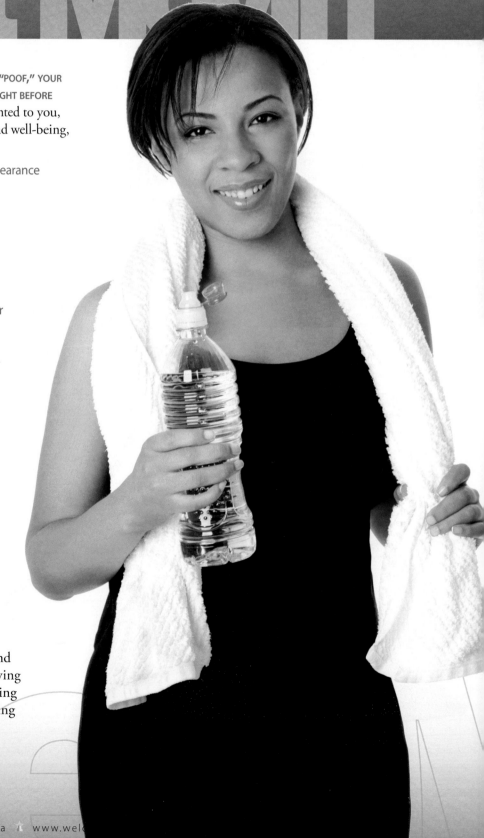

IMAGINE, JUST SNAP YOUR FINGERS AND "POOF," YOUR HEALTH AND FITNESS WOULD CHANGE RIGHT BEFORE YOUR EYES! If you had one wish granted to you, relating to your personal health and well-being, what would you wish for?

➤ A slimmer and trimmer appearance

➤ Vibrant energy

➤ Deep and relaxing sleep

➤ Lower stress

➤ More muscle tone

➤ Better flexibility

➤ Look and feel years younger

➤ All of the above

Wouldn't it be wonderful to snap our fingers and realize our deepest health and fitness desires? What if I told you that no matter what shape you are in right now, or how many times you may have tried to improve your health and well-being in the past, you are much closer than you think to turning your hopes into reality. In fact, you are just one step away from realizing your health and fitness wish. By reading this book, you'll discover seven simple moves that will dramatically impact your body and life—empowering you to get moving again, re-energizing and recapturing your health and fitness, and making your dreams come true!

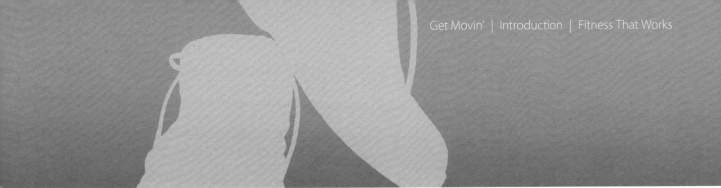

One Chapter—One Move

Throughout this book you will be introduced to a unique and practical approach to making fitness work. I will teach you how to select from seven simple "moves," which, when performed well, will make you stronger, physically younger, healthier, more productive and so much more! I will be introducing you to a new move each chapter; showing you why each move is crucial for your fitness and health and how easy it is to incorporate all seven moves into your daily routine.

Best of all, the seven moves have been designed in such a way that you can perform them between 9 to 5—at work—while you are on the phone, in a meeting, on the manufacturing line, on a break, or even while flying in a plane.

So what are the seven simple moves?

Move #1: Balance

Move #2: Reach

Move #3: Step

Move #4: Push-Pull

Move #5: Squat-Lift

Move #6: Twist

Move #7: Lunge

ADVANTAGES TO THE 7 SIMPLE MOVES

Increase your energy.

Decrease your stress.

Look and feel younger.

Learn to move well and more often.

Realize a slimmer and trimmer appearance.

Re-energize and re-capture your fitness.

Enhance your productivity.

Discover the moves that work best for you and your body.

Design an exercise program specific to your personality, needs and interests.

You will learn how performing each of these movements on a regular basis can help you reach your fitness potential. I will show you how you can use each move to assess your current and potential fitness level as well as how to track your progress. I'll also share proven programs and resources that match your personality and how you can incorporate each move.

You'll also be motivated by proven *Fitness That Works* tips throughout the book and introduced to those who have made fitness work—at work—and discover how you can do it, too.

I promise you, by adding the seven moves and tips found in this book to your life, your future fitness and health will change for good. Best of all, you'll make your fitness dreams and wishes come true!

Are you ready? Here we go!

SIMPLE MOVES MOVE MOUNTAINS

Scientific Support For SIMPLE MOVES!

Numerous studies show individuals who perform "simple moves" combined together as part of their daily work routine can decrease their risk of injury while improving strength, coordination, balance, work productivity and much more. For example:

A study published in the *Journal of Occupational Medicine* studied the impact that a "simple moves" program had on 443 firefighters—by testing them and providing specific training to enhance their trunk stability and strength along with flexibility. Researchers discovered that by using a simple "movement" program specific to their needs, the group reduced lost time due to injuries by 62% and the number of injuries by 42% over a twelve month period (as compared to a historical control group).

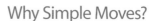

Get Movin'

Why Simple Moves?

Four years ago, my wellness practice was asked by a long-standing corporate manufacturing client of ours to create a fitness and productivity program for its employees. This company—a leader in the field of health and wellness—was experiencing decreased productivity, increased reports of fatigue and injuries, and slippage in job performances in key areas of the plant. Our wellness team's initial thought was to provide an exercise program after work. We were certain it would be a "slam-dunk" decision, as all the managers and supervisors understood that a fit employee is a much more productive employee. The challenge, as with most exercise regimens installed in the workplace, was the added time to an often already long day.

I had considered an exercise session during work hours, but this idea, while novel at the time, had many obstacles and "naysayers" who simply did not wish to change the status quo.

Some of the obstacles to holding work-day sessions included:

➤ High costs related to employees being away from their day-to-day job responsibilities.

➤ The exercise program would need to be a "no sweat" workout and performed in the issued uniforms, due to contamination protocols.

➤ All employees were to voluntarily participate.

➤ Because the program could only be voluntary, there needed to be a high enough adoption rate amongst a majority of employees for it to be considered a "fair and reasonable" use of resources.

Despite the obstacles, I still believed in the principles for exercise at work, and was able to convince management to agree to a pilot program to test the validity and impact of this idea.

When the program was underway, our wellness team began to analyze how the employees moved on a daily basis. This is when we noticed something shocking—**ALL** of the employees who were complaining about fatigue, muscular soreness, low productivity, etc., were **ALL** repeating the **same movements, every day, INCORRECTLY**!

PROOF IS IN THE PRODUCTIVITY

We wondered if a "simple moves" fitness break, involving easy-to-perform, replicable rejuvenating, non-sweat, balance, mobility, corrective, stretching and strengthening exercises performed on a daily basis would improve employee morale, presenteeism and/or productivity.

Our team partnered with Dr. Joe Leutzinger, president of the Academy of Health and Productivity Management and a leading expert in the field of worksite wellness, to research the effects of a "simple moves" approach during the work day. With a total of 141 participating employees, representing three departments from a California-based manufacturing company, we designed a 12-week "simple moves" intervention. Participants received five to fifteen minutes of "simple moves," non-sweat fitness breaks four days per week. To assess the ease, duplicability and affordability of this program, two of the sessions were provided by our wellness staff and the other two were delivered by trained volunteer employee ambassadors (who received monthly training, handouts of the exercises and support from our wellness team).

Using a validated questionnaire, all participants were then assessed before midway and at the end of the program. After the questionnaires were collected, the data analyzed by Dr. Leutzinger and his staff showed that there were statistically significant improvements in a number of areas with just a few minutes of "simple moves." These included:

➤ A desire for healthier living
➤ Improved morale
➤ Less "presenteeism"
➤ Expectations of the work unit to:
  – Exercise more   – Manage stress
  – Not smoke   – Work more productivity

"Results of the analysis indicate the program had a positive effect on participants and assisted them with starting or re-energizing their fitness routines. The program provides a tangible framework for helping individuals incorporate more physical activity into their daily routine. It also provides a viable mechanism for easing individuals into a more active daily fitness routine."

— Joe Leutzinger, PhD
President, Academy for Health and Productivity Management

We anticipated that some of the employees would have ergonomic and work-related issues, but we didn't realize **how many** of them were incorrectly performing their "simple movements" on a consistent, daily basis. These simple movements included motions such as: trying to maintain their balance when stepping over an object on the floor; walking up or down a flight of stairs; reaching up or down for something above their head or below their waist; lunging down when trying to tie their shoes; squatting to sit in a chair or pick up an object off the floor; lifting a box; or simply rotating their upper body when talking to someone behind them or moving a package. These simple movements, performed incorrectly every day, were creating a number of acute and immediate challenges for employees. We could see that if these were not corrected, the cumulative effect would lead to inevitable chronic issues that might jeopardize the employees' future health, fitness and livelihoods.

As a result of these findings, our team looked to experts in the field of occupational and physical therapy for solutions. One such expert was Gray Cook MSPT, a physical therapist and leading researcher in movement and sports performance. He took a systematic approach to working with athletes and focused on decreasing their incidence of injury while significantly enhancing performance. Mr. Cook discovered that through assessing human movement patterns and providing "corrective training" to combat any personal weaknesses or imbalances, an individual can consistently decrease their chances of injury and improve their performance.

According to Mr. Cook, **"just because someone has the ability for movement does not mean they have command of the movement. We must first learn to move well—then move more often."**

Get Movin'

Simple Moves = Big Results

Our wellness team thought that since you could decrease injury in elite athletes through simple, corrective movement training—then the workplace would be a breeze! So, we set out to create a program that not only retrained each employee to move correctly, but also helped them to positively impact their health, fitness and productivity. Because we had identified some key areas of poorly executed on-the-job movements that were impacting employees, we wanted to find corrective solutions. So, we began to look at other research related to "simple movements," both in and out of the workplace, making special note of primary movement patterns and any issues relating to the following areas:

➤ Stability, neuromuscular and proprioception training (or balance movements).

➤ Mobility/stretch training (or reach movements).

➤ Circulatory/Cardiovascular strengthening (or step movements).

➤ Functional training (or push-pull, squat-lift, twist, and lunge movements).

The scope of the research our team reviewed ranged from random populations to collegiate and professional athletes—and also to corporate settings. All the research we collected was from an array of disciplines related to fitness, physical therapy, occupational therapy, relaxation training, stress management, biomechanics and ergonomic training.

All of the studies we analyzed supported the idea that a "simple movement" program—if it's specific to one's needs and performed on a regular basis—can make a significant difference in the health, fitness, performance, productivity and life of any individual who participates.

After compiling all of our information and research, we then went to work putting together a "simple moves" program. Then we evaluated the impact of this program in our manufacturing client's work environment. We were thrilled at the response and the results!

To our surprise, we discovered that even if employees performed just a few of the "moves" well, they identified the following outcomes: "feeling better, moving more effectively and having a greater sense of well-being."

You've probably heard the saying: "You're only as strong as your weakest link." When this notion is applied to our physical fitness (and virtually all areas of our lives), this quote becomes a beacon of light that reveals a timeless principle. If there's the slightest weakness or the tiniest "crack" in one area related to our physical fitness, this weak link can ultimately mean the difference between:

➤ Optimal strength versus muscular weakness and injury;

➤ Robust energy and vitality versus debilitating fatigue;

➤ Lasting longevity versus premature aging; or

➤ Vibrant health versus chronic disease.

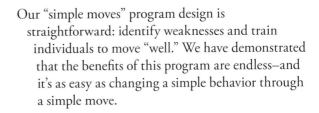

Our "simple moves" program design is straightforward: identify weaknesses and train individuals to move "well." We have demonstrated that the benefits of this program are endless–and it's as easy as changing a simple behavior through a simple move.

My goal for you is also simple—I want to help you move well and move often.

Right now, you're holding that program in your hands! *Fitness That Works: Simple Moves To Make Exercise Happen From 9 To 5* is ready for you!

What are we waiting for?…Let's get moving!

BEFORE YOU BEGIN—READ THIS…

Q: What's the best exercise for you?
A: The one you will do—and do well!

It's one thing to understand how simple moves can make a big difference in your life—but it's quite another to actually make it a part of your life. Before we dive into the seven simple moves, it's important to understand your options when personalizing any fitness program.

Personality has a lot to do with what you enjoy and ultimately what type of exercise program will work for you. When you're "making your moves" and planning your regular fitness routine, it's important to stick with a style of exercise you enjoy. For example, if you're more social, you may enjoy a fitness class as opposed to working out solo. Or, if you're self-disciplined and enjoy having time for yourself, you might enjoy running or walking alone. Knowing your strengths and potential weaknesses can help you select the moves, activity or fitness program that works best for you and fits your personality.

Get Movin'

Getting Started, Or Starting All Over Again? Five Steps For Fitness Success!

1 Know You Can Do It!
The first step to getting started and creating an active lifestyle is to begin believing that you can do it! No matter what your past experiences have been in getting or staying physically fit, or how many times you have tried and failed in the past…you have a choice to take responsibility for your future. Commit to taking positive steps to improve your fitness level—know you can do it!

2 Identify Weaknesses
The strongest and most successful athletes in the world are the ones who focus on improving their weaknesses, not their strengths.

When it comes to the success of your personal fitness, this statement was one of the key discoveries we made when reviewing the research about simple moves.

It is very important to identify any faulty movement patterns, muscle weaknesses, or conditioning challenges you have before beginning your personal fitness plan. This is for your safety, efficiency and overall progress. Throughout this book, at the end of each chapter, you will be given simple movement tests you can perform to help you identify your personal weaknesses. NOTE: If you would like to learn more about more advanced forms of fitness testing, see the resources and references section on page 150–151.

3 Identify Your Fitness Personality
Ask yourself, "What do I enjoy?" "What do I like?" "What is something I'll look forward to doing?" "What activity, workout or consistent 'moves' fit my personality?" Over the 20 years I have been working in the fitness field—especially in corporate settings—I have found that the most effective way to ensure your long-term success with any fitness endeavor is to first identify what you enjoy*. When you understand what makes you tick, what you like or what you don't like, you are much more likely to attempt and continue your exercise plan.

*You can take the "Fitness That Works Personality Quiz" on page 16 to determine what makes you tick!

4 Determine Your Goals
To incorporate "simple moves" every day and make fitness a regular part of your life, you'll have to be honest with yourself when identifying where you are now and where you want to be.

A Where do you want to be? What do you want to accomplish in the next year? What would you like to accomplish in the next three months, six months and the next year? Take a few moments to write down your specific long and short term goals relating to your health and fitness.

B What will help you reach your desired goals? Ask yourself this question as it relates to your fitness program, "What is one thing I am not doing right now that if I did start doing on a regular basis I KNOW would help me reach my desired fitness goals?"

For example: Is it scheduling your workouts or maybe getting an exercise buddy? Take some time to brainstorm the possibilities.

C What are you willing to do to reach your goals? If you think about your future personal fitness program, what obstacles will you need to overcome to help you get back or stay on track? What support systems can you put in place to help "coach" and support you to do the things you know are best for you?

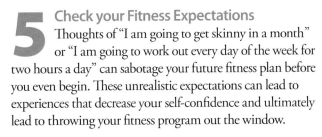

5 Check your Fitness Expectations

Thoughts of "I am going to get skinny in a month" or "I am going to work out every day of the week for two hours a day" can sabotage your future fitness plan before you even begin. These unrealistic expectations can lead to experiences that decrease your self-confidence and ultimately lead to throwing your fitness program out the window.

Instead of setting unrealistic goals and expecting perfection from yourself, begin by systematically "planning experiences" that you know you can achieve.

Instead of designing your future fitness program with the idea that you will exercise six days your first week (when you have not exercised in six months), begin by planning to review the suggestions in this book and start small.

Remember, you don't have to be perfect to be physically fit! If you miss an exercise session or were inactive for a short period of time, which will happen, don't beat yourself up with condemnation or punishment. Simply assess your lifestyle at the time, learn from it, forgive yourself and plan to get back into your new active lifestyle as soon as possible. Don't waste time beating yourself up…just get back to it!

Maintaining an active healthy lifestyle requires confidence, a good plan, persistence and most importantly, forgiveness! Put this all together and the future of your fitness looks very bright!

To further get to know your fitness personality, take the quiz on page 16. The Fitness That Works Personality Quiz, (adapted from the American Institute for Cancer Research Personality Quiz), is designed to help you identify what type of exercise personality you have—your Fitness That Works personality profile—and what simple moves are best for you. At the end of the quiz, you'll have the opportunity to score your results and learn more about what makes you tick from a fitness perspective. At the end of each chapter, you'll also discover customized "simple move" recommendations for your designated Fitness That Works Personality Profile.

Get Movin'

Fitness That Works Personality Quiz

Check the box on the left of the statement that best describes you.

1 **When I am at work, I usually perform my best when:**

☑ I am left to work on my own.		A
☐ I have the opportunity to work with a group to share our creative thoughts.		B
☐ I am given instructions but can come and go as I please.		C

2 **When thinking about exercise, I:**

☐ Can't wait to put on my walking shoes or lift weights.		A
☑ Really want to get moving but need a nudge to get fit and stay fit.		B
☐ It's tough for me to be consistent but enjoy it when I'm doing it!		C

3 **When I am active, I enjoy exercising:**

☑ Solo—by myself.		A
☐ As part of a team or class.		B
☐ With a buddy or maybe two.		C

4 **When I take part in exercise, I usually:**

☑ Plan and schedule the activity ahead of time.		A
☐ Participate when someone else arranges the activity or class.		B
☐ Make it happen on the fly and do something I'm in the mood for.		C

5 **When it comes to my motivation to exercise, I usually:**

☑ Want to lose weight, get in shape or improve my health.		A
☐ Enjoy having fun with friends and working out together.		B
☐ Am active because it's a nice day outside or I just feel like it.		C

6 **I enjoy activities that:**

☑ I set up and manage.		A
☐ Are led by a professional, team or group.		B
☐ Are adventurous, spontaneous and fun.		C

7 **Others see me as:**

☑ Self-disciplined and a leader.		A
☐ A team player.		B
☐ Fun loving and someone who goes along with a good idea.		C

RESULTS	A	B	C
Your Total: Check your quiz answers and add up the total number of corresponding "A's" "B's" and "C's" from the right-hand column.	6	1	
Your Profile: The highest total is the letter that matches your recommended Fitness That Works Personality Profile. What's yours? Write it down in the box provided.	**My Profile is:** A		

Why Should I Know My Fitness That Works Personality Profile?

It would be wonderful if there was one exercise program that worked for everyone, but since we all have different goals, interests and personalities, it takes some "trial and error" to make fitness work. Based upon your quiz results, if you scored higher in a designated area than another, you can speed up the process by learning more about your fitness personality and selecting from the proven tips listed under your personality profile.

(Note: Even though your main strengths/skills/interests may be focused in one area, everyone is different and not all profiles will be a perfect match all the time.)

A PROFILE A

If you scored higher in A's, you tend to be self-motivated. "A's" are individuals who tend to be decisive, independent, self-disciplined and results-driven, and pride themselves on reaching their established goals. Profile A individuals also prefer to exercise alone and participate in activities they can control and manage themselves, for example, walking, weight training or running. They excel when scheduling and planning their workouts and monitoring their own progress. This profile typically needs a nudge to get moving and prefers more details about "why" an exercise program is needed or beneficial, but once they have a plan in place, watch out!

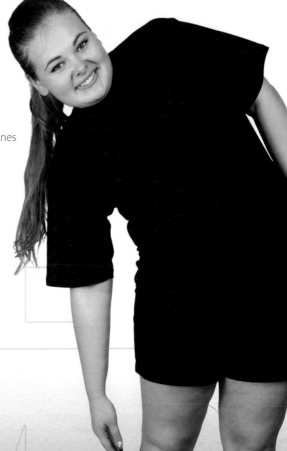

Strengths

➤ Enjoy working out alone—not overly dependent on others for fitness success

➤ Have the ability to challenge and motivate themselves

➤ Excel with setting goals and tracking personal progress

➤ Enjoy learning about health and fitness

➤ Do best with routines, structure and scheduling

Challenges

➤ Can lose interest in exercise if no challenge or goal is established

➤ Experience boredom or burnout due to getting stuck in the same exercise routines

➤ Can be afraid to try new exercise programs, which can lead to fitness plateaus

➤ Struggle with motivation if accomplishing goals or progress seems slow

➤ Overanalyze fitness programs

Tips And Recommendations

Profile A (Self-Motivated) individuals are most successful with:

➤ Setting monthly, quarterly and yearly fitness goals

➤ Signing up for an event such as a 5K Walk/Run or half-marathon

➤ Scheduling personal "exercise appointments" before the work week begins

➤ Keeping a workout journal to monitor progress

➤ Tracking fitness moves, workouts and activities using tools such as pedometers, online journals and/or fitness tracking software

➤ Hiring a personal trainer or having a workout buddy to help mix up routines

➤ Reading or viewing the latest fitness books and or DVDs

➤ Trying new moves* to vary their routine

(*See recommendations at the end of each chapter.)

Get Movin'

B PROFILE B

If you scored higher in B's you tend to be a support seeker. "B's" are individuals who thrive in social settings. They prefer exercising in groups, participating on teams, sharing fellowship, and energizing and encouraging others. Profile B individuals prefer incorporating physical activity and classes in their lives rather than working out alone. Profile B individuals enjoy a challenge as long as there are others to encourage and support their efforts.

Strengths

➤ Enjoy working out with others
➤ Are motivated to learn from instructors or trainers
➤ Like being pushed to higher levels of training
➤ Enjoy learning new activities and exercises
➤ Are socially oriented and find strength in numbers

Challenges

➤ Use exercise as a way to socialize, which can lead to inconsistency if friends leave the class or group
➤ Disappointment with class instructor or trainer can impact exercise adherence
➤ May have issues with over-training and injury

Tips And Recommendations

Profile B (Support Seeking) individuals are most successful with:

➤ Joining classes or recreational sports teams and clubs through work or community groups
➤ Doing challenging exercises during group or class workouts
➤ Social networking and posting fitness experiences and success
➤ Enlisting an exercise buddy to go to class or workout with
➤ Participating in corporate or community boot camps and group challenges
➤ Signing up for workout classes or personal training
➤ Trying new moves*, which can be performed with a group

(*See recommendations at the end of each chapter.)

C PROFILE C

If you scored higher in C's, you tend to be spontaneous. "C's" are drawn to activities, individuals, technology and environments that are engaging and fun, and those that provide an opportunity for spontaneity and self-expression. Profile C participants generally do not like structure, as they prefer not to have a schedule guide their exercise choices. Easily bored, Profile C individuals love to choose from an array of options and activities they can sample, such as recreational sports, fun fitness games or equipment. For a "C," the greater the variety, the better. Profile C individuals also enjoy challenging themselves with new activities that connect them to their sense of playfulness.

Strengths

➤ Enjoy a variety of activities (especially recreational games and sports)

➤ Typically their motivation is not impacted by a lack of results (e.g. losing weight)

➤ Exercise for the pure enjoyment, experience and fun of it

➤ Are generally good at a number of different types of activities or sports

➤ Are motivated by fun and/or different forms of movement

➤ Do best with spontaneity and various types of exercise

Challenges

➤ Do not like schedules or routines

➤ Lack of scheduling can lead to inconsistency

➤ Motivation to exercise can be negatively impacted by outside factors (e.g. bad weather or not being in the mood to exercise)

Tips And Recommendations

Profile C (Spontaneous) individuals are most successful with:

➤ Joining sports clubs or teams and competing on a seasonal basis, (e.g. Winter: Racquetball; Spring: Softball; Summer: Tennis; and Fall: Basketball)

➤ Experimenting with various fitness technologies, (e.g. fitness apps and digital or online workouts)

➤ Creating a fitness "toy box" at work or home, which is used to play with different types of exercise equipment, such as jump ropes, balance and medicine balls, stretch ropes, kettle bells and resistance bands

➤ Soliciting a buddy or two to join in various weekly, monthly or quarterly activities

➤ Rotating or "cross training" selections from the "Simple Moves" program*, so workouts are varied and intermixed

(*See recommendations at the end of each chapter.)

Now It's Time To Learn The Seven Simple Moves To Make Exercise Happen From 9 To 5

Balance

Life is like riding a bicycle. To keep your balance, you must keep moving.

—Albert Einstein

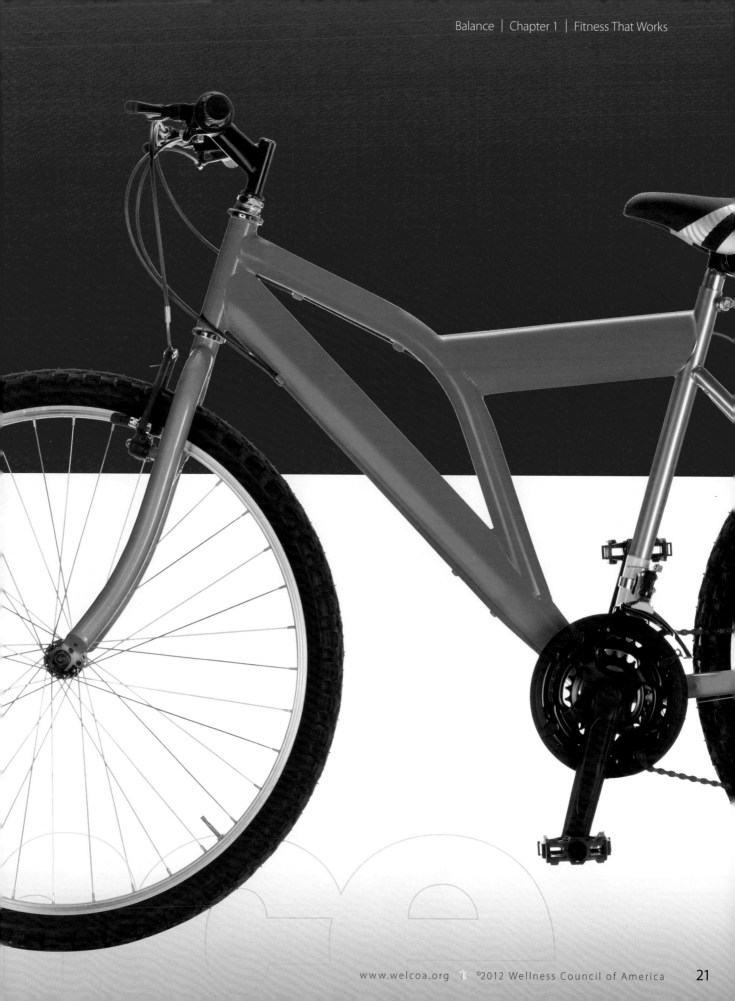

Balance

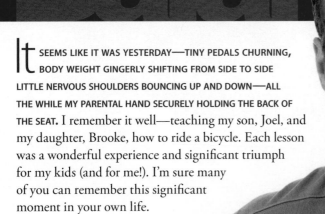

It SEEMS LIKE IT WAS YESTERDAY—TINY PEDALS CHURNING, BODY WEIGHT GINGERLY SHIFTING FROM SIDE TO SIDE LITTLE NERVOUS SHOULDERS BOUNCING UP AND DOWN—ALL THE WHILE MY PARENTAL HAND SECURELY HOLDING THE BACK OF THE SEAT. I remember it well—teaching my son, Joel, and my daughter, Brooke, how to ride a bicycle. Each lesson was a wonderful experience and significant triumph for my kids (and for me!). I'm sure many of you can remember this significant moment in your own life.

We owe this memory all to persistence, patience, and most importantly, learning how to balance. Without balance, we may have wanted to—even tried to—but ultimately would not have been able to ride that bike! Because it's been years since most of us learned how to ride a bike, we often take this simple movement and our sense of balance for granted. We rarely take time to think about how difficult it was to learn a new movement—let alone how important a strong sense of balance is to the quality and enjoyment of our lives.

In this first chapter, we will look closely at our first, most foundational simple move: Balance. Chapter 1 explores:

1 Different types of balance

2 Why balance is so important

3 How aging and inactivity impacts your balance

4 How to test your balance

5 Simple moves you can do to improve your balance

6 Recommended balance programs, tools and more

Brian: From "Spaz-im" To "Stud"— The Power Of Balance Training

Brian was a middle-aged truck driver who found himself in the doctor's office with significant pain and discomfort from an injured shoulder and wrist. Brian had injured himself when he fell while getting out of his truck, landing directly on his right arm and shoulder.

His family physician, Doctor James, listened as Brian shared what happened: "Doc, I don't know what's wrong with me. I just can't seem to find my footing! I keep stumbling and slipping. It started with a few trips, then a couple of spills, but I was always able to catch myself before really getting hurt. But this time, I just couldn't stop myself from falling right on the pavement—SMACK!" Doctor James looked at Brian's shoulder and wrist, and then performed some ear and eye examinations and other assessments. After ruling out inner ear and vision problems, Doctor James asked Brian to do some simple movement tests. After completing the tests, Doctor James asked Brian what his exercise and activity habits had been over the last few years. Brian replied: "Well doc, I just don't have the ability to exercise with my job. I am on the road all the time—I usually don't roll into a town until late at night and then I'm up early the next morning. Makes it tough to do any kind of exercise."

Doctor James asked, "When is the last time you exercised?"

"Well, I used to play softball on a regular basis, but it's been quite a while—maybe two or three years," Brian said. "Come to think of it, that's when I started noticing I couldn't hit very well and kept stumbling when running around the bases."

Doctor James smiled and said: "Brian, I believe your slipping and falling challenge is primarily due to a weakening of your balance systems."

"My what?!" shouted Brian.

"You see, your ability to balance your body—whether you are standing still or moving—is dependent upon your inner ear, vision and the intricate communication system between your brain, nerves, joints and muscles. If this communication system isn't used enough, it gets weak and the signals don't work as well—nor does your body respond as quickly when you need it to. Because you are sitting the majority of the day while driving, your muscles and joints have become weaker, and your communication system between your nervous system, brain and body has become sluggish and slower," noted Doctor James.

"Is it something I can fix?" asked Brian. Doctor James put his hand on Brian's shoulder, smiled and said, "Yes, absolutely it is something you can fix. You can retrain your communication system to work automatically—the way it used to when you were younger and active. I am going to give you some simple movements you can use on a daily basis to retrain your body and your brain to work together to help improve your balance."

Doctor James treated Brian for his dislocated shoulder and sprained wrist, and then prescribed some simple moves to help him improve his balance and strength. Three months later, Brian's shoulder and wrist were completely healed and he had faithfully been doing his simple moves to strengthen his balance. Brian had made the time to do his simple moves outside of his truck at every rest stop on road trips. Not only did Brian find his footing, he felt stronger and more confident again, and even joined a softball league that played twice a week! (Oh, and by the way, Brian led that team in homeruns last season!)

Balance

What Is Balance?

The dictionary defines balance as "a physical equilibrium or stability produced by even distribution of weight on each side of the vertical axis." Whew! That's a mouthful! While it sounds fancy, this definition is a bit limited and too technical-sounding for my taste. I prefer to view balance as one's ability to maintain a center of gravity.

Our body will constantly try to find a "center" or equilibrium at all times, whether we are standing still or moving. There's an intricate interconnection between the brain, inner ear, nervous system and your muscles, ligaments and tendons—and they're all working together in perfect harmony to help your body stay upright.

BRAIN TRAIN

The simple skill of balancing your body when standing on one foot, climbing out of a truck, or even walking is dependent upon an intricate communication system between your brain, nervous system, muscles, ligaments and tendons. It's called "proprioception" and is your body's unconscious ability to interpret messages about the position of your body and movement. This amazing ability allows you to sense which muscles to activate and contract to achieve a desired motion or position—like raising your arm to scratch your head—without even thinking about it. Unfortunately, if we don't actively use this system, it becomes weaker and slower, and movement becomes more difficult.

By practicing balance training, movement patterns and skills (like riding a bike or driving a car) that once seemed daunting will become simple and automatic, requiring little thought to execute. By training your balance, you can improve proprioception, coordination, strength, agility, and master more complex movements, (think of an athlete catching a ball with one foot in the air, one on the ground and the rest of his/her body parallel to the field). Balance is the foundation to all human movement. Your ability to balance your body impacts all of your daily activity as well as your ability to perform more complex movements.

LOSING YOUR BALANCE

Believe it or not, your natural ability to balance your body (when standing or moving) begins to decline after the age of 25! How fast it declines depends upon how much you move your body and practice balancing. By practicing balance training, you can keep this necessary skill in peak shape.

Two Types Of Balance

STATIC BALANCE. Your ability to maintain your center of gravity in a non-moving position, such as sitting upright on the edge of your chair or standing in line, is highly dependent on strong stabilizing structures in your body, including your ligaments, tendons and muscles.

> **BENEFIT ➤** The number one benefit to strong static balance is an ability to prevent falling when in a non-moving position—without it you wouldn't be able to sit upright, stand, or shift your weight from one foot to the other. Another important benefit is a strong and healthy posture. By strengthening key stabilizing ligaments, tendons and muscles, you can improve your body posture and alignment significantly—helping you look stronger, younger and healthier.

DYNAMIC BALANCE. Your ability to maintain balance while moving, such as when you're walking, stepping over an object, jogging, jumping, cycling or dancing, is ultimately dependent upon your body working in sync with your brain, vestibular system (vision and inner ear), nervous system, muscles and ligaments.

> **BENEFIT ➤** A strong sense of dynamic balance enhances your ability to be successful in any movement activity—from the simplest, to the most complex. Dynamic balance allows you the ability to tie your shoes without falling, change direction when jumping over a puddle, and run and turn to catch a fly ball in the World Series.

How Inactivity And Aging Impacts Balance

Have you ever heard the phrase, "If you don't use it, you'll lose it?" Well, when it comes to your balance—this most certainly rings true. Research indicates that as we grow older and less active, our ability to balance our body—both when still or in motion—diminishes significantly.

According to the Centers for Disease Control and Prevention, one of every three Americans over the age of 65 falls each year. Elderly trips, falls and spills are primarily related to an inability and weakening of both static and dynamic balance.

According to Debra Rose, Professor of Kinesiology and Co-director of the Center for Successful Aging at California State University-Fullerton, "As we grow older, our balance and mobility becomes compromised, often for a variety of reasons: lack of lower body strength, altered sensory or motor function, certain medications or diagnoses, or a combination of these variables. When a fall occurs, it often creates such a fear that the older adult becomes even less active. Of course, this lack of physical activity creates even more mobility problems—making the likelihood of falls even more pronounced. It's a downward spiral."

While a number of aging-related issues such as inner ear problems, vision challenges and mobility issues contribute to falls, the good news is that research indicates you can do something about this. Through simple moves and balance training, you can practice and significantly improve your balance skills to reduce the risk of falling—while bringing health, vitality and balance back to the body.

MUSCULAR BALANCE

Technically, there is also one additional aspect to balance that we need to consider—and that's muscular balance. Much of our physical health is dependent upon the health, strength, flexibility and balance of our muscles. Without a proper balance of strength, flexibility and endurance between opposing muscles, such as the front of the leg (quadriceps) and the back of the leg (hamstrings), we are very susceptible to injury, fatigue and weakness.

Muscular Balance = Equilibrium Between Muscles

This is absolutely crucial in avoiding short term and long-term injury and enhancing performance in all static and dynamic movements.

Balance Moves & Balance Tests That Work At Work
Try the moves and tests on the following pages to help improve your balance!

It's time to improve your...
Balance

It's time to move...

Balance Move #1: Standing One-Leg Balance

Here's a great simple move to help you improve your balance (specifically your static balance). The best part is, you can do this while on break at work, in the office, or even when combing your hair!

➤ **GET READY**

You'll need a flat, non-slip surface to stand on and a timing device (such as a watch) to keep track of your time.

➤ **GET SET**

Standing tall and upright with your feet together, place your hands on your hips.

➤ **GO**

When you are ready, raise the right knee up, towards your waist-line, while maintaining balance on the left standing leg. Next, place your right foot near the inside of your left knee- and hold.

Next, raise up on the ball of the standing left foot and raise both arms out to the side, raising your arms and hands to shoulder level. Try to maintain balance for up to 30 seconds.

Repeat these steps, three times on each leg.

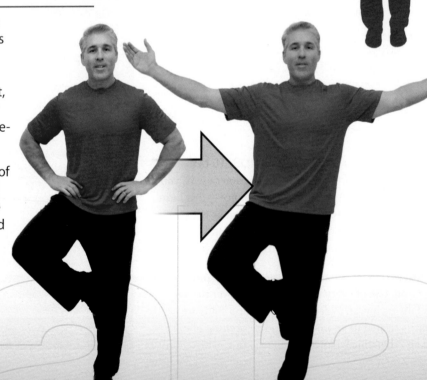

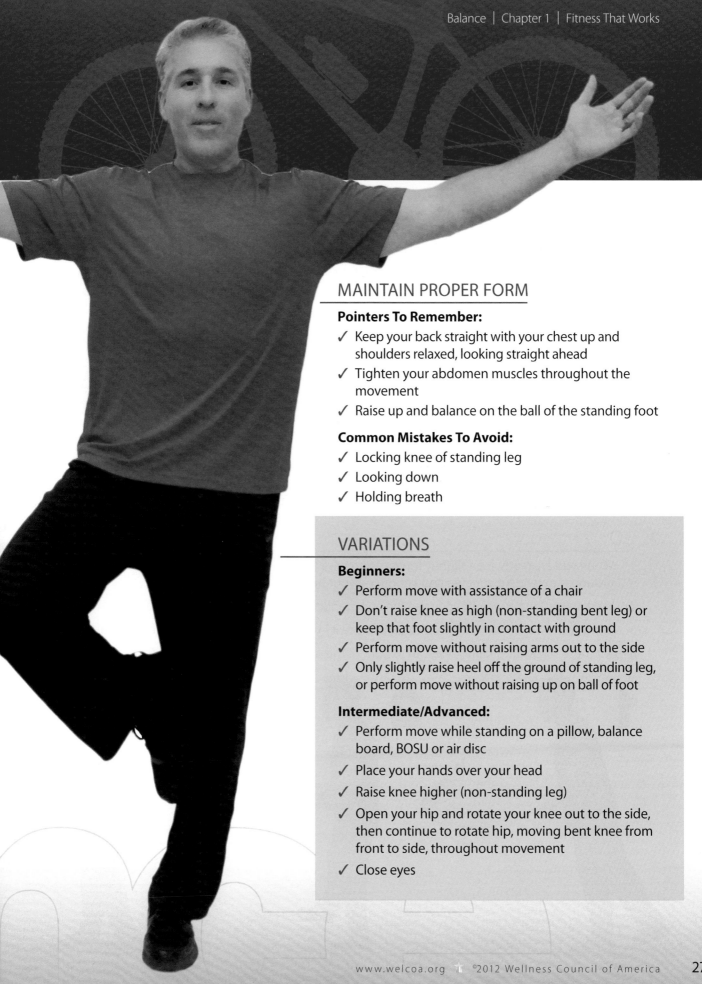

MAINTAIN PROPER FORM

Pointers To Remember:

✓ Keep your back straight with your chest up and shoulders relaxed, looking straight ahead

✓ Tighten your abdomen muscles throughout the movement

✓ Raise up and balance on the ball of the standing foot

Common Mistakes To Avoid:

✓ Locking knee of standing leg

✓ Looking down

✓ Holding breath

VARIATIONS

Beginners:

✓ Perform move with assistance of a chair

✓ Don't raise knee as high (non-standing bent leg) or keep that foot slightly in contact with ground

✓ Perform move without raising arms out to the side

✓ Only slightly raise heel off the ground of standing leg, or perform move without raising up on ball of foot

Intermediate/Advanced:

✓ Perform move while standing on a pillow, balance board, BOSU or air disc

✓ Place your hands over your head

✓ Raise knee higher (non-standing leg)

✓ Open your hip and rotate your knee out to the side, then continue to rotate hip, moving bent knee from front to side, throughout movement

✓ Close eyes

It's time to improve your…

Balance

Now, try this move…

Balance Move #2: Moving Balance—Walk The Line

Here's a great simple move to help you improve your overall balance (especially your dynamic balance), and one you can also perform throughout your work day—especially when you are walking from one area to another.

➤ GET READY

All you'll need is a flat, non-slip surface to walk on.

➤ GET SET

Standing tall and upright, place one foot in front of the other, heel to toe—then raise your hands and arms out to the side, at shoulder level.

➤ GO

1. When you are ready, lean slightly forward and raise the back foot behind you—slightly off the ground—extending your leg and tightening your buttocks.

2. Next, balance your weight and raise the non-standing leg and foot out to the side.

3. Bring your non-standing foot around and place it in front of the standing foot, heel to toe.

Repeat these steps, alternating one foot in front of the other up to 10 times for each foot.

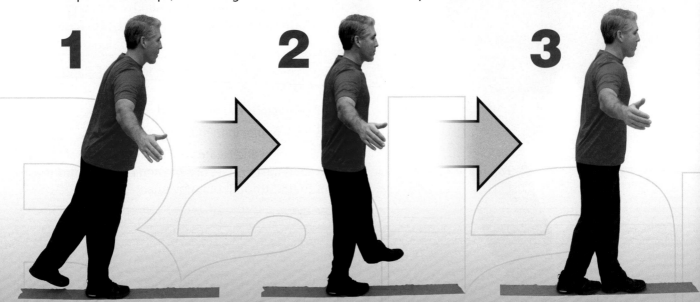

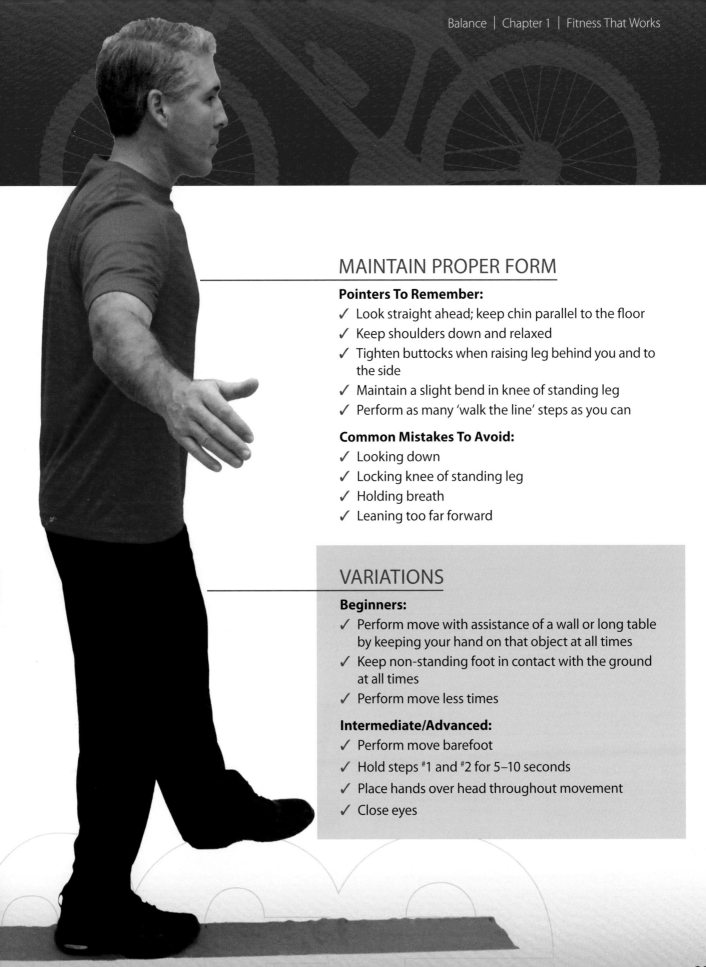

MAINTAIN PROPER FORM

Pointers To Remember:
✓ Look straight ahead; keep chin parallel to the floor
✓ Keep shoulders down and relaxed
✓ Tighten buttocks when raising leg behind you and to the side
✓ Maintain a slight bend in knee of standing leg
✓ Perform as many 'walk the line' steps as you can

Common Mistakes To Avoid:
✓ Looking down
✓ Locking knee of standing leg
✓ Holding breath
✓ Leaning too far forward

VARIATIONS

Beginners:
✓ Perform move with assistance of a wall or long table by keeping your hand on that object at all times
✓ Keep non-standing foot in contact with the ground at all times
✓ Perform move less times

Intermediate/Advanced:
✓ Perform move barefoot
✓ Hold steps #1 and #2 for 5–10 seconds
✓ Place hands over head throughout movement
✓ Close eyes

It's time to test your…

Balance

Now it's time to test your balance! How balanced are you? Take a moment to find out…

Balance Test #1: The Stork Balance Test

This test measures your ability to stand in a non-moving position while standing on one leg and on the ball of your foot. This test is a good indicator of how you're doing when it comes to static balance.

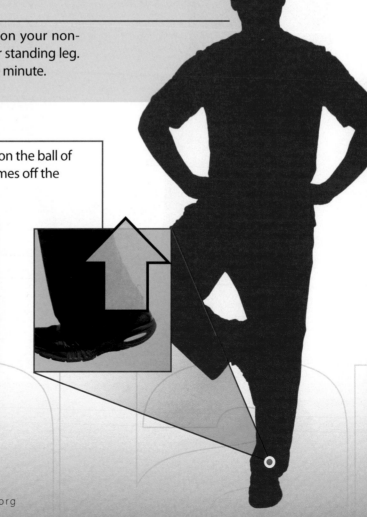

➤ **GET READY**

You'll need a flat, non-slip surface to stand on, a stop watch or clock, a pencil or pen and this book to score your results. Also, be sure to remove your shoes before beginning your test.

➤ **GET SET**

Position your hands on your hips and position your non-supported foot against the inside knee of your standing leg. You can practice the test for approximately one minute.

➤ **GO**

When you are ready, raise your heel to balance on the ball of your foot. Begin timing as soon as your heel comes off the ground.

➤ **FINISH**

Stop timing when:

✓ Hands come off the hips

✓ The non-supported foot loses contact with the knee

✓ The heel of the supported foot touches the floor

✓ The supporting foot swivels, moves or hops in any direction

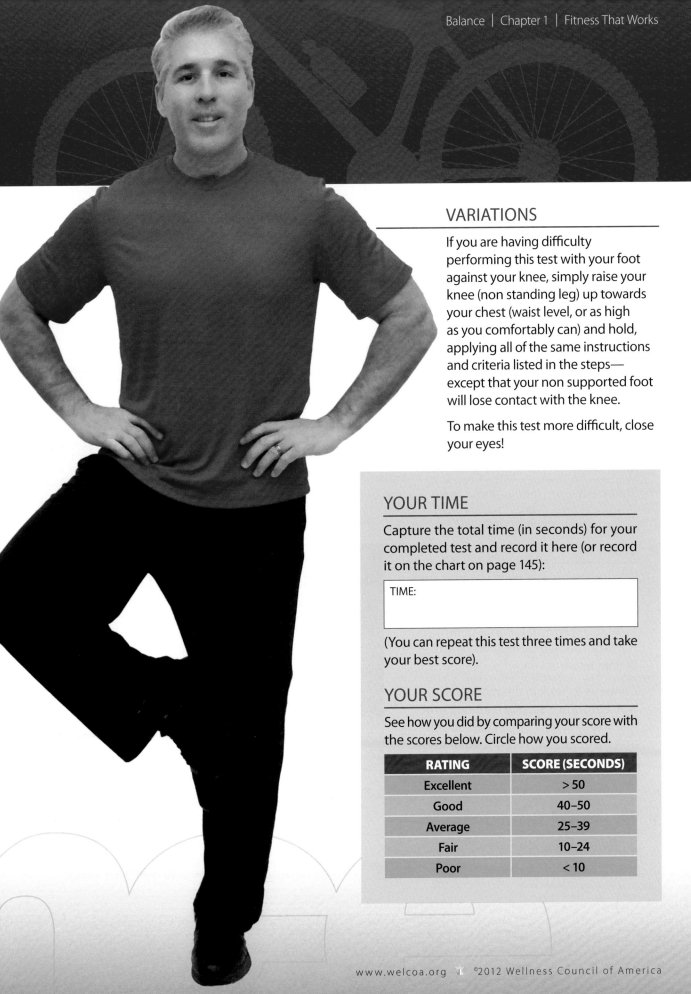

VARIATIONS

If you are having difficulty performing this test with your foot against your knee, simply raise your knee (non standing leg) up towards your chest (waist level, or as high as you comfortably can) and hold, applying all of the same instructions and criteria listed in the steps—except that your non supported foot will lose contact with the knee.

To make this test more difficult, close your eyes!

YOUR TIME

Capture the total time (in seconds) for your completed test and record it here (or record it on the chart on page 145):

TIME:

(You can repeat this test three times and take your best score).

YOUR SCORE

See how you did by comparing your score with the scores below. Circle how you scored.

RATING	SCORE (SECONDS)
Excellent	> 50
Good	40–50
Average	25–39
Fair	10–24
Poor	< 10

It's time to test your...

Balance

Here's another simple test you can take to see how dynamically balanced you are...

Balance Test #2: Walking The Line Test

This test measures your ability to move and balance your body at the same time while stepping with one foot in front of the other (heel to toe) on an imaginary or real line.

➤ GET READY

You'll need a flat non-slip surface, preferably a line or masking tape to represent a straight line, a pencil or pen and this book to score your results. This test can be performed with or without shoes.

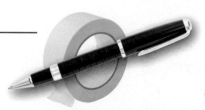

➤ GET SET

Stand with both feet together in front of the beginning of a straight line (or imaginary).

➤ GO

While keeping your hands by your sides at all times, place your left foot on the line and then your right foot in front of it, touching heel to toe. The heel of your right foot should be touching the toes of your left foot.

Continue to walk in this manner, watching your feet and counting how many total steps you can take. (If you are in a small area, count 10 total steps and turn around and walk back.)

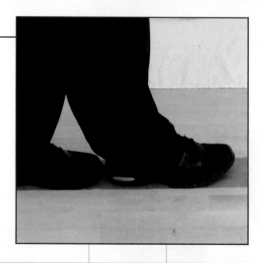

➤ TERMINATE THE TEST IF...

✓ You cannot keep your balance on the line

✓ You have to stop walking to balance yourself

✓ You are not able to touch heel to toe

✓ You have to use your arms to balance yourself

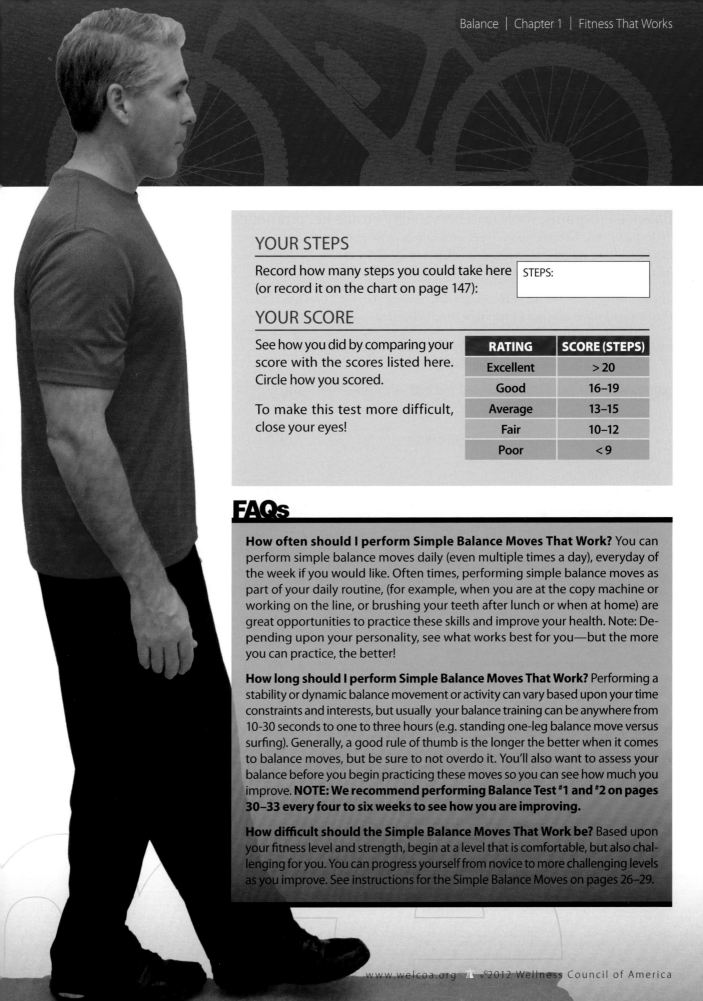

YOUR STEPS

Record how many steps you could take here (or record it on the chart on page 147):

STEPS:

YOUR SCORE

See how you did by comparing your score with the scores listed here. Circle how you scored.

To make this test more difficult, close your eyes!

RATING	SCORE (STEPS)
Excellent	> 20
Good	16–19
Average	13–15
Fair	10–12
Poor	< 9

FAQs

How often should I perform Simple Balance Moves That Work? You can perform simple balance moves daily (even multiple times a day), everyday of the week if you would like. Often times, performing simple balance moves as part of your daily routine, (for example, when you are at the copy machine or working on the line, or brushing your teeth after lunch or when at home) are great opportunities to practice these skills and improve your health. Note: Depending upon your personality, see what works best for you—but the more you can practice, the better!

How long should I perform Simple Balance Moves That Work? Performing a stability or dynamic balance movement or activity can vary based upon your time constraints and interests, but usually your balance training can be anywhere from 10-30 seconds to one to three hours (e.g. standing one-leg balance move versus surfing). Generally, a good rule of thumb is the longer the better when it comes to balance moves, but be sure to not overdo it. You'll also want to assess your balance before you begin practicing these moves so you can see how much you improve. **NOTE: We recommend performing Balance Test #1 and #2 on pages 30–33 every four to six weeks to see how you are improving.**

How difficult should the Simple Balance Moves That Work be? Based upon your fitness level and strength, begin at a level that is comfortable, but also challenging for you. You can progress yourself from novice to more challenging levels as you improve. See instructions for the Simple Balance Moves on pages 26–29.

Balance

Balance Programs, Tools And Personality Profile Recommendations

To improve your balance, you can perform simple movements such as those mentioned on pages 26–29. Or you can select from various recommended balance programs and tools that we recommend based upon your Fitness That Works Personality Profile.

The following chart is a list of recommended balance activities. (See specific recommendations for your Fitness Personality Profile checked in the right hand columns).

Fitness Personality Profile—My Personality Profile Is

▼ Check three that are the most appealing to you.

BALANCE ACTIVITIES/EXERCISES	PROFILE A	PROFILE B	PROFILE C
☐ Simple Moves: One Leg Balance (See page 26–27)	✓	✓	✓
☐ Simple Moves: Moving Balance (See page 28–29)	✓	✓	✓
☐ Pilates		✓	
☐ Tai Chi		✓	
☐ Yoga/Dynamic Stretching Classes		✓	
☐ TRX Training	✓	✓	
☐ Boxing Classes		✓	
☐ Ballet		✓	
☐ Dance Classes (Ball Room, Zumba)		✓	
☐ Stability Ball Training	✓	✓	✓
☐ BOSU Training	✓		
☐ Air Disc Training	✓		
☐ Jumping rope	✓		✓
☐ Walking or running barefoot	✓		✓
☐ Bowling			✓
☐ Trampoline	✓		✓
☐ Horse shoes			✓
☐ Bocce Balls		✓	✓
☐ Golf	✓	✓	✓
☐ Surfing			✓
☐ Skateboarding			✓
☐ Softball/baseball		✓	✓
☐ Racquet Sports (Tennis, Badminton, Racquetball)		✓	✓
☐ Fencing		✓	
☐ Gymnastics	✓	✓	
☐ Martial Arts Training	✓	✓	
☐ 4–3–2–1 Fitness Training (See page 148–149)	✓	✓	✓

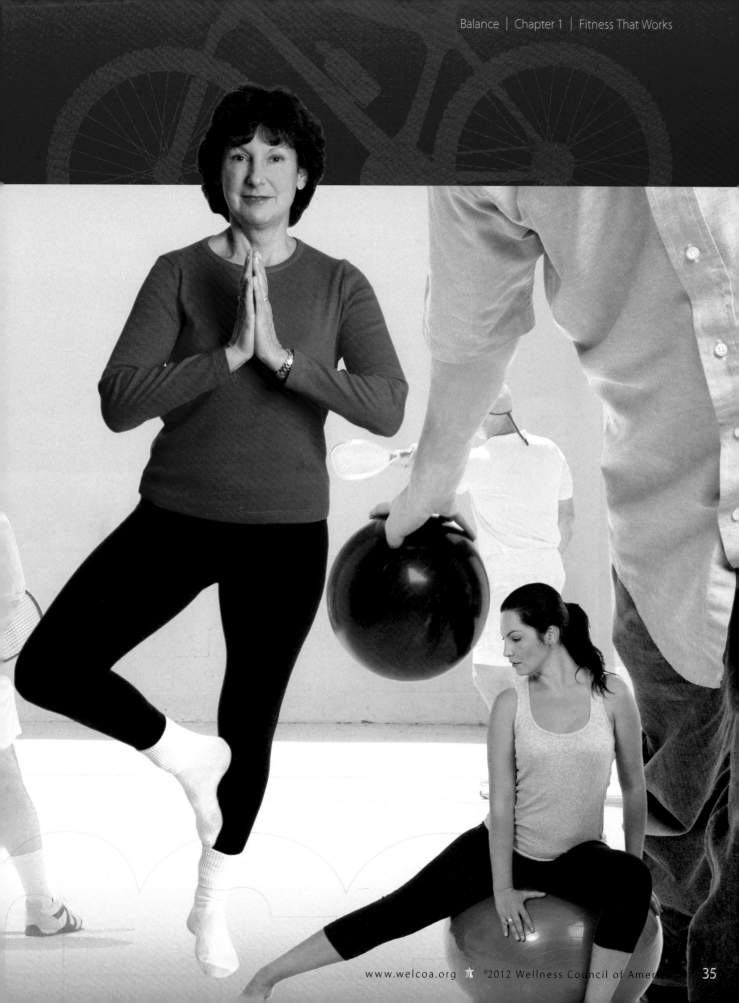

Reach

> *"Keep your feet on the ground and keep reaching for the stars."*
>
> —Casey Kasem

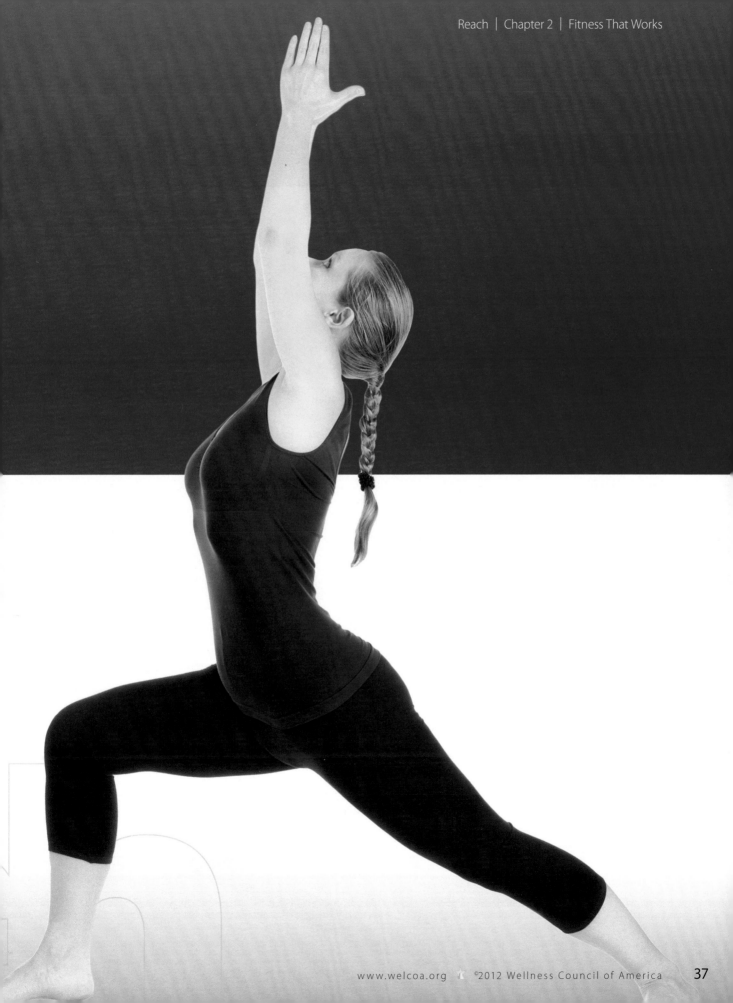

Reach

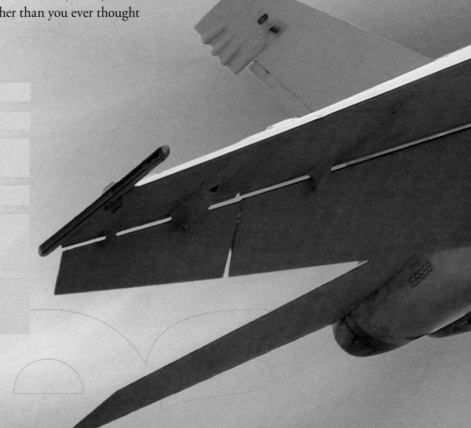

In 1912, THE FIRST COMMANDING OFFICER OF THE CANADIAN ROYAL FLYING CORPS (RFC), COLONEL FREDERICK SYKES, CHALLENGED HIS MEN TO COME UP WITH A MOTTO THAT WOULD INSPIRE, MOTIVATE AND INSTILL COURAGE WHEN CONFRONTED WITH DIFFICULTY AND ADVERSITY IN BATTLE. Two junior officers came up with the inevitable historic slogan, an ancient Latin phrase, "sic itur ad astra," which is loosely translated: "reach for the stars." To this day, a slightly different version of this phrase, "through struggles to the stars," has remained the proud battle cry of The Royal Canadian Air Force.

For most of us, "reach for the stars" has been a saying with which we are familiar and encouraged by in our own lives. In this chapter, I want to challenge you to adopt a slightly shorter version of this motto: "Reach." You'll be amazed how this simple word and move will inspire you—and bring healing, health and hope back to your body and life.

In this chapter we will look at our second move, reach, and how it can take your physical fitness higher than you ever thought possible—maybe even to the stars.

We will explore:

1   What is reach?

2   Why reach is so important

3   How inactivity and aging impacts your reach

4   How to test your reach

5   Simple moves you can do to improve your reach

6   Recommended reach programs, tools and much more

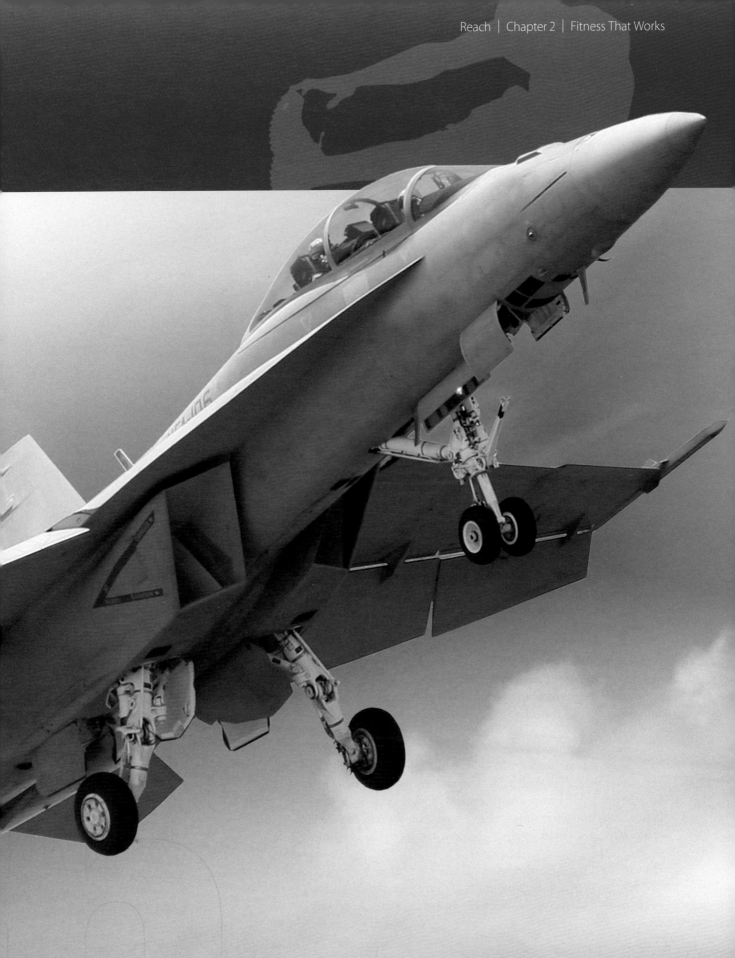

Reach

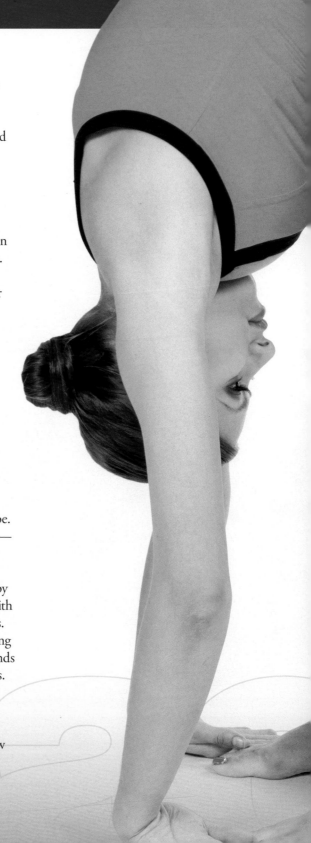

Can You 'Reach' Your Toes?

"Well, can you mom?" Jane wasn't sure how to take this challenge from her 14 year old daughter, especially since it had been years since she had performed the splits or really challenged herself like she had back in her cheerleading days. "Sure I can!" Jane exclaimed to her daughter. "Just watch."

Jane hesitantly put her feet together, took a deep breath and slowly began to descend to the floor, trying to reach down and touch her toes. To her surprise (and her daughter's laughter and smirks), she could only reach slightly beyond her knees. Jane tried again and then again, going a little further each time, but it wasn't going to happen. Her toes seemed miles and miles away. That night, as Jane thought about her inability to reach the ground, a wave of sadness came over her. She began to think about how her fitness had "slipped away" and how this small "failure" mirrored the majority of her life.

For Jane, over the last few years, everything she tried seemed to end in disappointment. She was struggling. Overweight, low energy, sore aching muscles, and fighting to reach goals she had set for herself months and even years ago, she was slowly giving up on her dreams, her hopes and herself. Little did Jane realize, her inability to reach the ground was just what the doctor (or should I say daughter) ordered.

Jane realized that night, for the first time in a long time, that her mobility, flexibility, fitness and life was not where she wanted it to be. She made a commitment to faithfully work on reaching the ground— and her goals. This time though, Jane decided to do it differently.

This time, she committed herself to making daily changes that, inch by inch, she hoped would eventually yield big results—beginning first with her reach. She set a goal and made the commitment to touch her toes. So, Jane decided to stretch when she was in the shower, or when waiting in line, or at work after sitting for two hours. She'd take a few seconds every chance she got to slowly reach down and try to touch her toes.

During this time, Jane also began to set other goals to improve her diet, get to bed earlier and start walking again. Slowly, she began to see progress towards reaching all of her goals. After a few months of performing this simple move and practicing her reach, Jane slowly began to get closer to her goal and ultimately her toes. On a day she will forever remember, she finally reached the ground and grabbed her toes!

Along with the benefit of improved mobility and flexibility, Jane would have never realized that a simple challenge to reach down and touch her toes would ultimately lead to so much—helping her to lose 30 unwanted pounds, alleviating her lower back pain, lowering her stress and realizing the energy, strength, fitness, hope and smile of a teenage cheerleader once again.

Reaching her goal of touching her toes was a turning point for Jane. She realized that goals she once thought were far away or had passed her by were now within reach. Jane shared, "You should have seen my daughter's face when I reached down and grabbed my toes! I think she was more proud of me than I was!"

This simple move, for Jane, served as a reminder and a symbol that she could accomplish any goal to regain her youth, vitality and passion for experiencing life again-all it took was a little "reach."

REMEMBER WHEN?

What games, recreational activities or sports did you enjoy participating in when you were a child or teenager? Take a moment to think back and remember what game, sport or physical activity you loved to do. Jot down how you felt when you were participating in these games, sports or activities:

When you read or hear the words, "FITNESS & EXERCISE," what do you feel? Take a moment and jot down your thoughts, feelings and ideas. What emotions come to the surface when you think about moving your body?

On a scale of 0-10, how would you rate your desire to exercise? Take a moment and chart your excitement level when it comes to moving your body on a regular basis:

0 ------1------- 2--------3--------4---------5--------6--------7------ 8 -------9------ 10

I Can't Stand It   **I'm Okay With It**   **I Love It**

What Is Reach?

Reach is our ability to stretch towards something, which we do when we need to touch, grasp, hold or obtain an object. Figuratively, the definition for reach can be used to refer to most anything you would like to obtain or achieve. Physically, your ability to accomplish simple daily tasks such as reaching down and picking up the morning newspaper, or reaching out to grasp your driving wheel when steering your car, or to open a door or shut a window, or reaching up to take down a box from a top shelf are all examples of the physical power of the move, reach.

BRAIN TRAIN

Reach = Flexibility + Stability + Mobility

Put into more technical terms, reach involves your body's ability—and more specifically, the joints of your body—to be mobile, giving you the strength, stability and flexibility to extend or move in a full range of motion. Experts would agree that to reach effectively, you need to have flexible muscles to allow you to stretch, which is what we call flexibility. But, reach also involves two other dimensions: stability and mobility. Stability relates to a strong support system—ligaments, tendons, bones and fascia (a web like sheath running from the bottom of your feet to the top of your head)—which provides your body with the necessary structure to hold you up and prevent your body from moving in a direction you don't want it to go. Mobility, on the other hand, is your ability to move and control a particular joint or body part (e.g. neck, shoulder, arm, hand, torso, hip, leg and/or ankle), contracting your muscles to take that body part through a full range of motion (such as reaching down and touching your toes).

The Goal Of Reach

The goal with the move of reach is simple: to increase and improve your flexibility, stability and mobility to the major joints of your body. This will help you to physically reach further with your body—and ultimately, your health and fitness goals.

Three Ways To Improve Your Reach

STATIC STRETCH. The most common form of stretching that will help improve your reach is called a "static stretch." Static stretching involves reaching or extending a muscle or muscle group to a point of tension (or its furthest point) and holding for a period of time, usually 15-30 seconds. A good example of this type of stretching is a standing or sitting toe touch.

The goal of static stretching is varied. It can be used to assess tightness in a particular muscle group or joint, or to promote relaxation and decrease stress—but is primarily used to elongate the muscle to increase flexibility and range of motion. The latest research demonstrates that the best time to perform static stretching movements is after physical activity/exercise or sporting events to increase blood circulation and deliver much needed oxygen and nutrients to sore muscles—as well as to increase flexibility and range of motion of muscles and joints.

BENEFITS ➤ Static stretching improves your reach by lengthening muscles and it offers many benefits, including:

- Increasing blood circulation;
- Sending needed nutrients and removing waste products to and from cells;
- Increasing joint mobility;
- Improving body posture and symmetry;
- Decreasing pain;
- Minimizing muscular soreness after physical activity/ exercise; and
- Assisting in decreasing stress.

DYNAMIC STRETCHING. A recently popular form of stretching to improve your reach that is gaining vast acceptance in the professional athletic and training world is called "dynamic stretch." Unlike static stretching, dynamic stretching encourages "active stretch movements" that gradually and safely use momentum, exaggeration or action to gently propel a muscle into an extended range of motion (think of a slow and controlled cabaret leg kick). This type of movement increases body temperature and blood circulation to the muscle or muscle group without holding it to a point of tension, which—as the latest research has uncovered—properly prepares muscles and joints for future activity, exercise or sport. Think of dynamic stretch movements as "moving stretches." Examples of dynamic stretches are shoulder arm circles or walking lunges or leg kicks.

BENEFITS ➤ Dynamic stretch movements increase body temperature, blood circulation, fluid production, balance, body awareness, stability, strength and joint range of motion, as well as properly prepare the body for peak performance and activity or exercise-reducing injuries. Current research demonstrates this form of stretching is best performed before a sporting event or physical activity/ exercise.

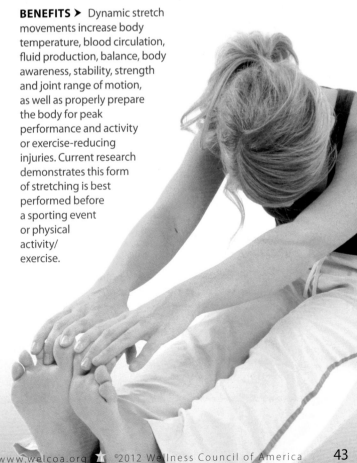

Reach

BRAIN TRAIN:

We've all been there—sitting for long hours in the same position and our back, shoulders and/or neck begin to feel like a bunch of tightly wound, knotted rubber bands— what we call kinks—that are ready to snap. To help alleviate this common physical ailment, researchers are now uncovering new treatments, methods and devices which have been found to not only relieve sore aching muscles, but also improve flexibility, mobility and range of motion. Recently, researchers have begun to understand the missing link to effective movement and treatment, and have found it all connects to fascia—literally! Fascia is a sheath-like connective webbing, which provides structure and support to the body, wrapping in and around muscles, tendons, ligament, nerves and organs. A good example of this is if you have ever cut through a piece of meat or prepared a turkey—when taking the skin off you'd notice a white colored sheath and tissue lying between the skin and the muscle. This is the fascia. What researchers are now beginning to understand is that fascia connects the entire body from head to toe, helping us move fluidly. Over time, however, as we grow older or as a result of inactivity, poor posture, overuse or injury, our fascia acts like a "patch" or "knot" in the muscle—and can create connective adhesions or "trigger points," limiting muscle blood supply, movement and leaving us to compensate in other muscles and joints.

Do you feel like your muscles are a bunch of "knots and kinks?" Stretching by itself may not be the only treatment to help you improve your reach. You may want to try and get the "knots and kinks" out first. A variety of therapies have been discovered to release or "untie" these adhesions, allowing the muscles and joints to move more freely. Here are some of the treatments that have been found to be beneficial:

✓ **Active Release Therapy** is a patented soft tissue and movement massage technique which helps with challenges related to fascia, muscles, tendons, ligaments and nerves.

✓ **Massage** comes in many different forms and techniques (for example, Deep tissue, Myofascial Release, Sports Massage, Shiatsu, Accupressure and Trigger Point Therapy are just a few). All are treatments which manipulate skin and "knead" muscles and or connective tissue (fascia, tendons and ligaments) to improve function, mobility or flexibility. Massage can also be used to promote relaxation and improve overall health and wellness.

✓ **Self Massage** is one of the fastest growing forms of getting rid of the "kinks." Self-massage is also known as "self myofascial exercise or treatment." Unique devices such as foam rollers (a cylindrical piece of hard or soft foam) and foam balls (tennis ball shaped, but structurally similar to foam rollers), are used to roll out tired and sore muscles. Therapeutic sticks—a hard or softer plastic stick shaped in different angles and sizes— are also handy tools, allowing you the ability to roll out knotted tissue and aching muscles. All of these devices are becoming common tools in therapeutic, collegiate and professional training rooms and are used both before and after exercise to reduce muscular soreness, improve flexibility, mobility and enhance your reach.

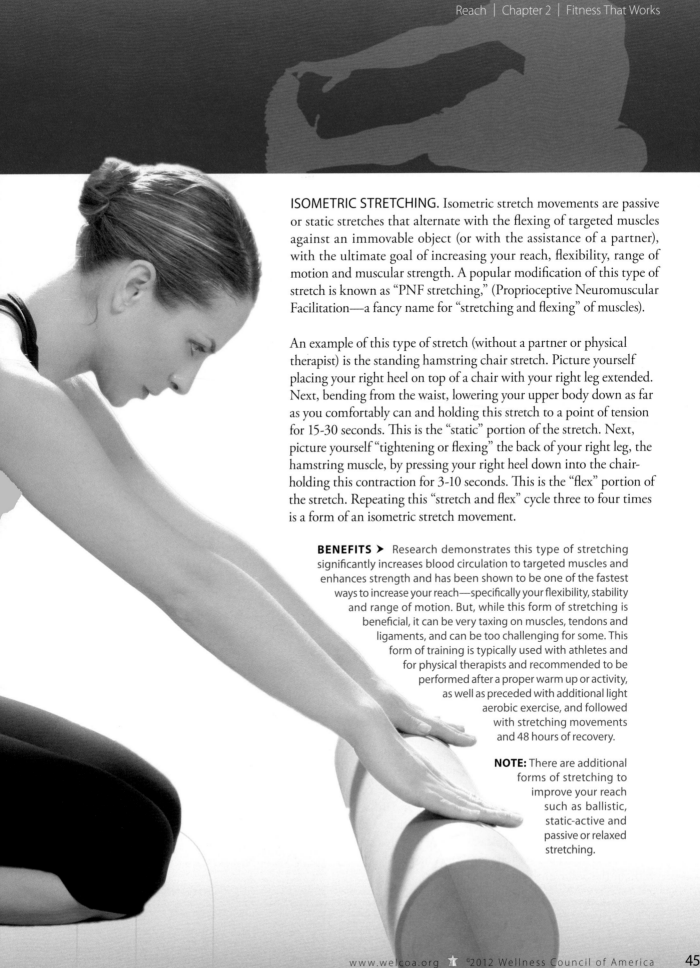

ISOMETRIC STRETCHING. Isometric stretch movements are passive or static stretches that alternate with the flexing of targeted muscles against an immovable object (or with the assistance of a partner), with the ultimate goal of increasing your reach, flexibility, range of motion and muscular strength. A popular modification of this type of stretch is known as "PNF stretching," (Proprioceptive Neuromuscular Facilitation—a fancy name for "stretching and flexing" of muscles).

An example of this type of stretch (without a partner or physical therapist) is the standing hamstring chair stretch. Picture yourself placing your right heel on top of a chair with your right leg extended. Next, bending from the waist, lowering your upper body down as far as you comfortably can and holding this stretch to a point of tension for 15-30 seconds. This is the "static" portion of the stretch. Next, picture yourself "tightening or flexing" the back of your right leg, the hamstring muscle, by pressing your right heel down into the chair-holding this contraction for 3-10 seconds. This is the "flex" portion of the stretch. Repeating this "stretch and flex" cycle three to four times is a form of an isometric stretch movement.

BENEFITS ➤ Research demonstrates this type of stretching significantly increases blood circulation to targeted muscles and enhances strength and has been shown to be one of the fastest ways to increase your reach—specifically your flexibility, stability and range of motion. But, while this form of stretching is beneficial, it can be very taxing on muscles, tendons and ligaments, and can be too challenging for some. This form of training is typically used with athletes and for physical therapists and recommended to be performed after a proper warm up or activity, as well as preceded with additional light aerobic exercise, and followed with stretching movements and 48 hours of recovery.

NOTE: There are additional forms of stretching to improve your reach such as ballistic, static-active and passive or relaxed stretching.

Reach

"You're Not In Kansas Anymore!" How Inactivity And Aging Impacts Your Reach

Do you remember the scene from the classic movie, *The Wizard of Oz*, when Dorothy and Scarecrow—on their way to the Emerald City—narrowly escape the talking, angry apple trees? After ducking and running away, do you remember what happened next? They come upon a statue of a figure that mumbles, "Oil!" Dorothy says, "Why, it's a man. A man made out of tin!" Scarecrow interjects, "I think he said, 'Oil can!'" Dorothy and Scarecrow ask the Tin Man where he wants to be oiled first and he says, "My mmmouth." The Tin Man struggles to talk, but then exclaims, "Me-me-mmmy, my, my goodness. I can talk again! Oh, oil my arms please—oil my elbows. Oh! Oh!" After a glorious time of freeing his limbs, the Tin Man was able to finally move. Dorothy and Scarecrow set the Tin Man free!

Many of us can relate to the plight of the Tin Man. Feeling rusty, stuck and unable to do simple movements that were once very fluid and easy to perform, but are now difficult and even painful. How many of us feel like we are stuck, immobile and in need of an oil can to lubricate our rusty joints?

According to the American Academy of Orthopedic Surgeons, inactivity and aging are two of the greatest challenges when it comes to maintaining or improving our mobility, flexibility and reach.

As we age, researchers point out that our muscles, ligaments and tendons become weaker, tighter and shorter. To compound this problem—weaker, tighter muscles leave already tight joints in a precarious place. With unwanted weight and strain now displaced on the weak joint, increasing discomfort leaves muscles tighter and more susceptible to injury. If that wasn't enough, add to this the common breakdown in cartilage, the "kinks" or trigger points that are created when muscle fibers adhere to one another and prevent the fibers from moving effectively, and to top it all off, a decrease in the body's production of a needed joint lubrication called synovial fluid—the typical wear and tear that our joints experience over the years leaves many without the desire or the ability to move.

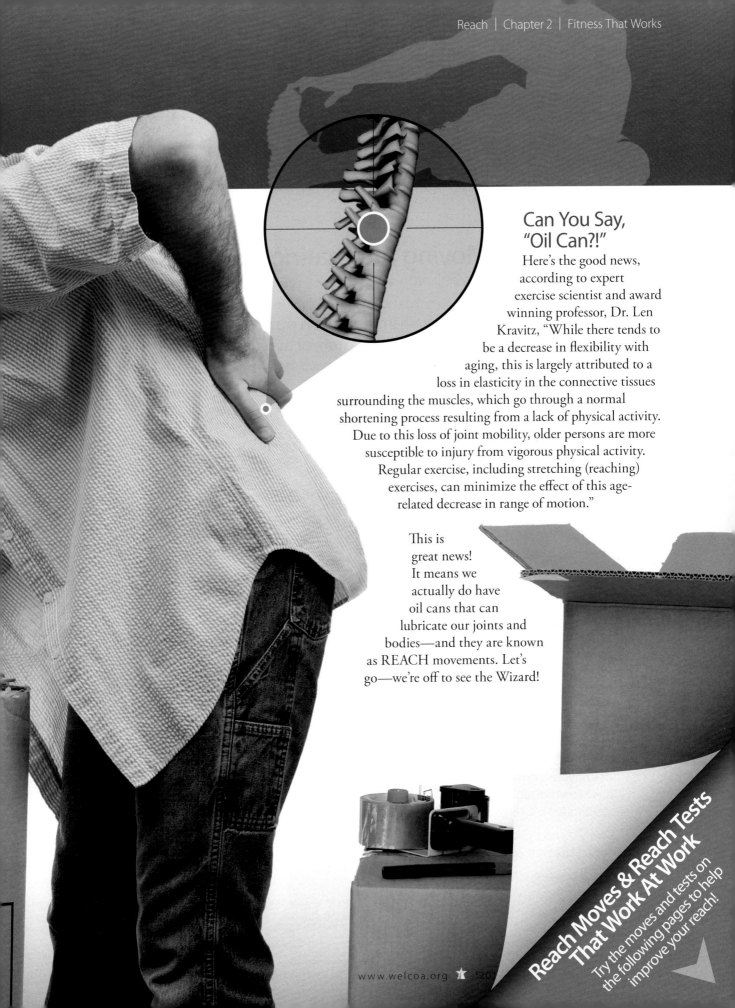

Can You Say, "Oil Can?!"

Here's the good news, according to expert exercise scientist and award winning professor, Dr. Len Kravitz, "While there tends to be a decrease in flexibility with aging, this is largely attributed to a loss in elasticity in the connective tissues surrounding the muscles, which go through a normal shortening process resulting from a lack of physical activity. Due to this loss of joint mobility, older persons are more susceptible to injury from vigorous physical activity. Regular exercise, including stretching (reaching) exercises, can minimize the effect of this age-related decrease in range of motion."

This is great news! It means we actually do have oil cans that can lubricate our joints and bodies—and they are known as REACH movements. Let's go—we're off to see the Wizard!

Reach Moves & Reach Tests That Work At Work

Try the moves and tests on the following pages to help improve your reach!

It's time to improve your…

Reach

It's time to move…

Reach Move #1: Moving Alternating Toe Touch

Here's a great simple move to help you improve your reach (specifically your Dynamic Reach)—helping to increase mobility, stability and flexibility for your upper and lower back as well as your hamstrings. This is a move you can do in front of your desk or even in the office in front of the coffee machine (OK maybe not, but you can do it most anywhere).

➤ GET READY

All you'll need is a flat, non-slip surface to stand on.

➤ GET SET

Standing upright, place your feet hip-width apart, with your legs straight and hands by your sides.

➤ GO

1. Take a small step forward (approximately 6-12 inches) with your right foot. Next, balance your weight and raise the non-standing leg and foot out to the side.

2. Slowly bend forward at your waist, rotating your torso, while reaching down with your left hand, trying to touch the toes of your right foot. Go down as far as you comfortably can and hold this position for 2-4 seconds.

3. Slowly stand upright and return to step 1. Repeat the motion to the other side.

Repeat these steps alternating legs four to six times each.

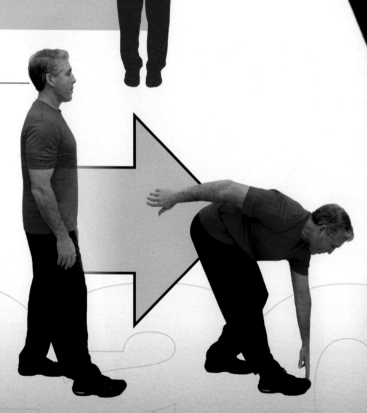

MAINTAIN PROPER FORM

Pointers To Remember:

✓ Move slowly and under control
✓ Bend at the waist, keeping your back straight
✓ Reach down and stretch until there's slight tension, but not pain
✓ Exhale as you lower down to reach toes
✓ Keep front leg being stretched straight and back leg bent

Common Mistakes To Avoid:

✓ Rounding your back
✓ Bouncing or jerking to reach toes
✓ Bending knees too much
✓ Holding breath
✓ Locking knees

VARIATIONS

Beginners:

✓ Keep the toes of the front foot on the ground throughout movement
✓ Use a chair for support
✓ Keep supportive hand on thigh throughout movement for additional support
✓ Don't go down as low

Intermediate/Advanced:

✓ Raise the toe towards the shin of the foot you are reaching toward
✓ Raise the back, non-stretched leg off the ground as you reach towards your toes— Note: keep the toes of the front foot on the ground
✓ Hold the stretch for a longer duration

It's time to improve your…

Reach

Now, try this move…

Reach Move #2: Shoulder Arm Circles

Here's one of my favorite simple moves to increase the range of motion and mobility in the shoulder joint—one of the most common areas of muscular tightness, weakness and inflexibility. I call this move "Shoulder Arm Circles." You may remember a form of this movement when you were younger, from warming your arms and shoulders up before playing a sport or game.

➤ GET READY

This move, which can be done anywhere, serves as a natural oil can, lubricating tight shoulder joints.

➤ GET SET

Stand upright, with your feet shoulder-width apart, knees slightly bent and your arms extended out to your sides, raised to shoulder level and palms facing the floor.

➤ GO

1. Begin to make small forward circular motions (about one foot in diameter) with your hands and arms in a controlled and slow fashion. Perform 10 times.

2. Now, begin to increase the size of your shoulder arm circles by progressing to medium to larger circular motions, until you are reaching as far forward and back as you comfortably can (i.e. above your head and below your hips). Perform 10 times.

3. Next, repeat the motion, by following steps 1 and 2, only reverse the motion, moving arms and hands in a reverse or backward motion.

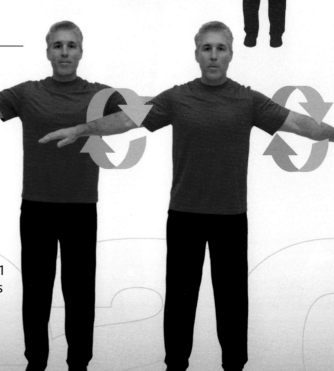

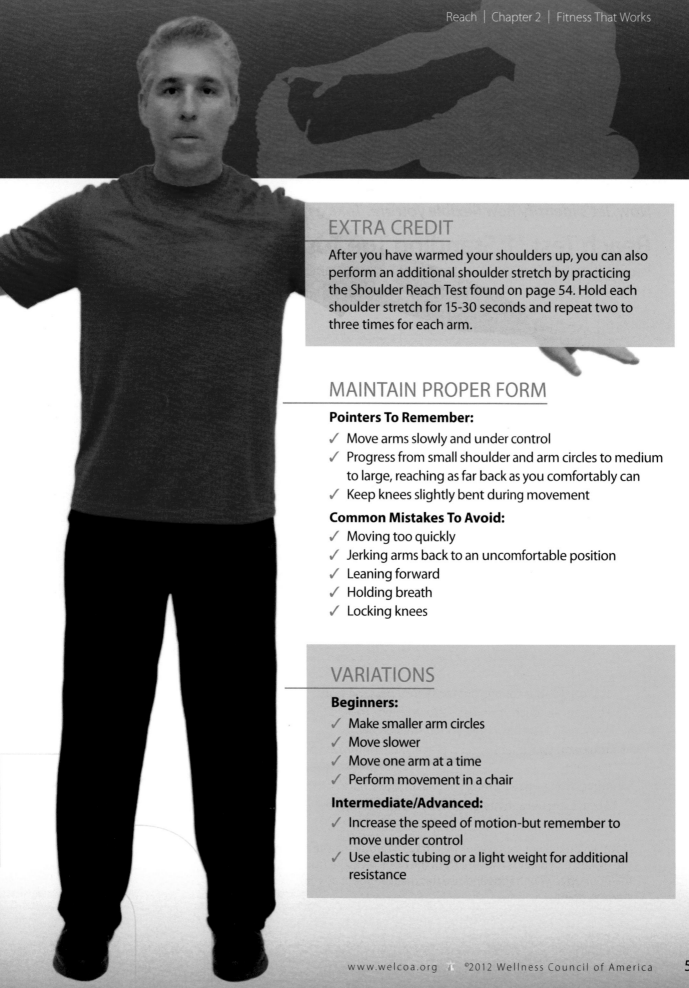

EXTRA CREDIT

After you have warmed your shoulders up, you can also perform an additional shoulder stretch by practicing the Shoulder Reach Test found on page 54. Hold each shoulder stretch for 15-30 seconds and repeat two to three times for each arm.

MAINTAIN PROPER FORM

Pointers To Remember:

✓ Move arms slowly and under control
✓ Progress from small shoulder and arm circles to medium to large, reaching as far back as you comfortably can
✓ Keep knees slightly bent during movement

Common Mistakes To Avoid:

✓ Moving too quickly
✓ Jerking arms back to an uncomfortable position
✓ Leaning forward
✓ Holding breath
✓ Locking knees

VARIATIONS

Beginners:

✓ Make smaller arm circles
✓ Move slower
✓ Move one arm at a time
✓ Perform movement in a chair

Intermediate/Advanced:

✓ Increase the speed of motion-but remember to move under control
✓ Use elastic tubing or a light weight for additional resistance

It's time to test your…

Reach

Now, let's identify how flexible you are. Take a moment to find out…

Reach Test #1: Standing Toe Touch

Having flexible muscles helps prevent injuries and increases range of motion. This test measures the flexibility of your lower back and hamstring muscles (back of the leg).

➤ **GET READY**

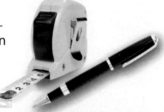

You'll need a flat, non-slip surface to stand on, a pencil or pen and this book to score your results. Also, it is recommended to remove your shoes before beginning your test.
Optional: Ruler or tape measure.

➤ **GET SET**

Stand upright, with your feet tight together, legs straight and hands on your thighs (palms down).

➤ **GO**

Slowly and under control, start the test by bending forward at your waist, reaching down with your hands trying to touch your toes. Make a mental note of where you were able to reach.

➤ **FINISH**

The test stops when:

✓ You can grab or touch your toes—You pass the test!

✓ You cannot touch your toes—No problem, make a mental note and compare your results below.

✓ You bend your knees—Keep practicing to improve your flexibility.

✓ You experience discomfort or pain in lower back— Always stop an activity or exercise if you feel pain or discomfort.

Note: If you did not touch your toes, have a buddy measure the distance your fingertips are from the floor. Measure from the floor up to your hands and use this measurement as your starting point.

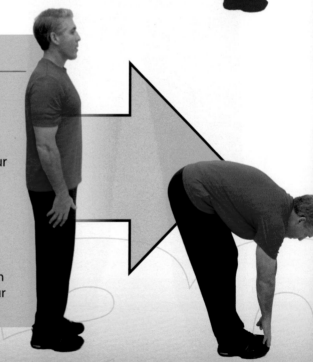

VARIATIONS

We strongly recommend warming your muscles up before performing this or any static stretch move. Also, If you have lower back problems, we recommend not participating in this test and/or performing a variation of this test, as follows.

The Seated Chair Toe Touch
Seated in a chair, with one leg extended, reach forward with both hands, bending from the waist, trying to reach/ touch your toes.

YOUR SCORE

Use the scale below or measure the distance that your hands are from your toes.

RATING	SCORE
Excellent	Grabbing toes
Good	Touching toes
Average	Touching top of foot
Fair	Touching top of ankle
Poor	Touching middle to lower shin

It's time to test your…

Reach

Now, it's time to take a look at your mobility as it specifically relates to your shoulders…

Reach Test #2: Shoulder Reach Test

This is a simple test to determine the mobility and flexibility of your shoulders.

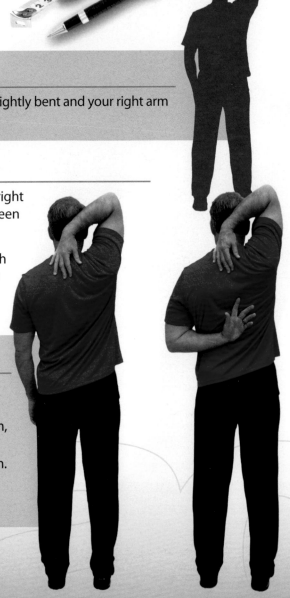

➤ GET READY

You'll need a flat, non-slip surface to stand on, a pencil or pen and this book to score your results.

Optional: Ruler or tape measure and a partner to measure your results.

➤ GET SET

Stand upright, with your feet shoulder width apart, knees slightly bent and your right arm in the air (as if you were asking a question).

➤ GO

Start the test by bending your right elbow, and with your right hand hanging behind your head, place your palm in between your shoulder blades.

Next, reach around your back with your left arm—and with the palm of your left hand facing away from your back, try to touch the fingers of your left hand with the fingers of your right hand.

➤ FINISH

The test stops when:
- ✓ You can touch your fingers together—You pass the test!
- ✓ You cannot touch your fingertips together—No problem, make a mental note and compare your results below.
- ✓ You experience discomfort or pain in the shoulder region.

Note: Switch hands and perform the test for the opposite shoulder.

VARIATIONS

If you'd like, you can have a buddy measure the distance between your fingertips by aligning your fingers and measuring the distance between the tips of your middle fingers. If you can touch your fingertips together, then your score is 0. If you cannot touch your fingertips then measure the distance between your fingertips as a negative score (for example, 1 inch = –1). If your fingertips overlap, then measure the distance as a plus score (for example, 1 inch = +1). You can perform this test two times and take your best score.

YOUR SCORE

Use the scale below or measure the distance that your hands are from your toes.

RATING	SCORE
Excellent	Fingers are overlapping
Good	Fingers are touching
Fair	Fingers are not touching, but are less than two inches apart
Poor	Fingertips are greater than two inches apart

Reach

FAQs

Depending on the form of the reach move that is chosen, the latest research points to performing stretches at specific times and in a specific fashion for best results.

How often should I perform Simple Reach Moves That Work? If you are doing static or dynamic movements, you can perform reach moves daily—even multiple times a day—every day of the week. But if you are performing isometric stretches, it is recommended that you give your body 48 hours in between sets to properly recover. You can even perform the Simple Reach Moves starting on page 48 at work (in the office or break room), or at home (in the shower like Jane!). **Note:** Depending upon your personality, see what works best for you, but the more you can practice reach moves—especially if they are static or dynamic—the better.

How long should I perform Simple Reach Moves That Work? Performing a static, dynamic or isometric stretch, class, move or activity can vary based upon time constraints and interests, but usually your reach training can be anywhere from 15–30 seconds to one to three hours (e.g. Alternating Toe Touch move versus a Karate class). Remember, regardless of the type of reach or stretching you choose to do, always warm up properly. Don't overdo it (yes, even with stretching you can do too much—especially if it is isometric). Also, be sure and assess your reach before you begin practicing these moves so you can see how much you improve. **Note: It is recommended to perform Reach Tests #1 and #2 on pages 52–55 every four to six weeks to see how you are improving.**

How difficult should the Simple Reach Moves That Work be? Based on your fitness level, flexibility and goals, you should begin at a level that is comfortable, but also challenging for you. You can progress yourself from novice to more challenging levels as you improve. See instructions for the Simple Reach Moves That Work on pages 48–51.

Since there are a few different types of stretching to improve my reach, what should I be mindful of? See the chart below for a breakdown of what, when and how to perform your stretches to improve your reach.

Types of Stretching	How Often?	Best time to perform?	How long?	How many times?
Static Stretches	Perform daily or even multiple times during the day	After physical activity or warm-up to help reduce muscle soreness and increase flexibility	Hold to a point of tension or stretch for 10-30 seconds	Upper and lower body, 2-3 times per muscle group
Dynamic Stretches	Daily	Before activity or event primarily use as a warm-up	Repeat movements 4-10 times	Full body, 2-3 times per muscle group
Isometric Stretch Movements	Every other day	After activity or event	Alternate "Stretch and Flex" by holding the stretch for 15-30 seconds and the flex for 3-10 seconds	Upper and lower body, 2-3 times per muscle group

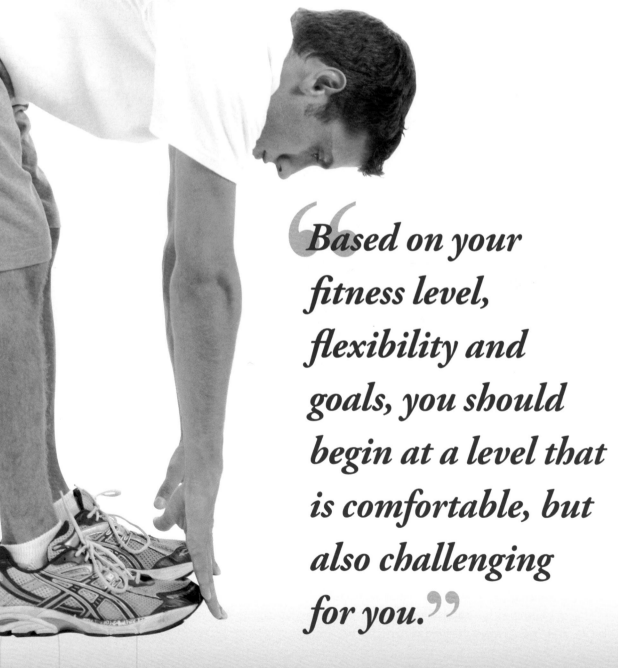

"**Based on your fitness level, flexibility and goals, you should begin at a level that is comfortable, but also challenging for you.**"

Reach

Reach Programs, Tools And Personality Profile Recommendations

To improve your reach, you can perform simple movements such as those we mentioned on pages 48–51. Also, based upon your Fitness That Works Personality Profile, you can select from the various recommended programs and tools below to help you with your reach. In the following chart, you'll see a list of recommended reach activities. (See specific recommendations for your Fitness Personality Profile checked in the right hand columns).

Fitness Personality Profile—My Personality Profile Is

▼ Check three that are the most appealing to you.

REACH ACTIVITIES/EXERCISES	PROFILE A	PROFILE B	PROFILE C
☐ Simple Moves-Moving Alternating Toe Touch (See page 48–49)	✓	✓	✓
☐ Simple Moves-Shoulder Reach (See page 50–51)	✓	✓	✓
☐ Pilates	✓	✓	
☐ Pilates Reformer	✓	✓	
☐ Tai Chi	✓	✓	✓
☐ Dynamic Stretching Classes (e.g. Yoga)		✓	
☐ Stability Ball Stretching	✓		✓
☐ Stretching with Resistance bands	✓		
☐ Ballet		✓	
☐ Dancing (e.g. Break Dancing, Hip Hop, Modern, Swing, Belly, Flamenco and Latin)		✓	✓
☐ Martial Arts (e.g. Aikido, Judo, Jujutsu, Kendo, Karate, Kung Fun, Mixed Martial Arts, Jeet Kune Do, Taekwondo)	✓	✓	✓
☐ Gymnastics	✓	✓	✓
☐ Rock Climbing			✓
☐ Parkour			✓
☐ Olympic Weight Lifting	✓		
☐ Stretch Station	✓		✓
☐ Self-Massage-Foam Roller/Balls/Sticks	✓		✓
☐ Stretch Straps	✓		✓
☐ Back Inversion Table	✓		
☐ Flexi-Bar (at home and classes)	✓	✓	✓
☐ Active Release Therapy	✓	✓	✓
☐ Massage (e.g. Deep Tissue, Myofascial Release, Sports Massage, Shiatsu, Acupressure or Trigger Point Therapy)	✓	✓	✓
☐ PNF Stretching	✓		
☐ Golf	✓	✓	✓
☐ Racquet Sports (e.g. Tennis, Racquetball, Badminton)		✓	✓
☐ Fencing		✓	
☐ Wrestling (Greco and Freestyle)	✓	✓	✓
☐ 4–3–2–1 Fitness Training (See pages 148–149)	✓	✓	✓

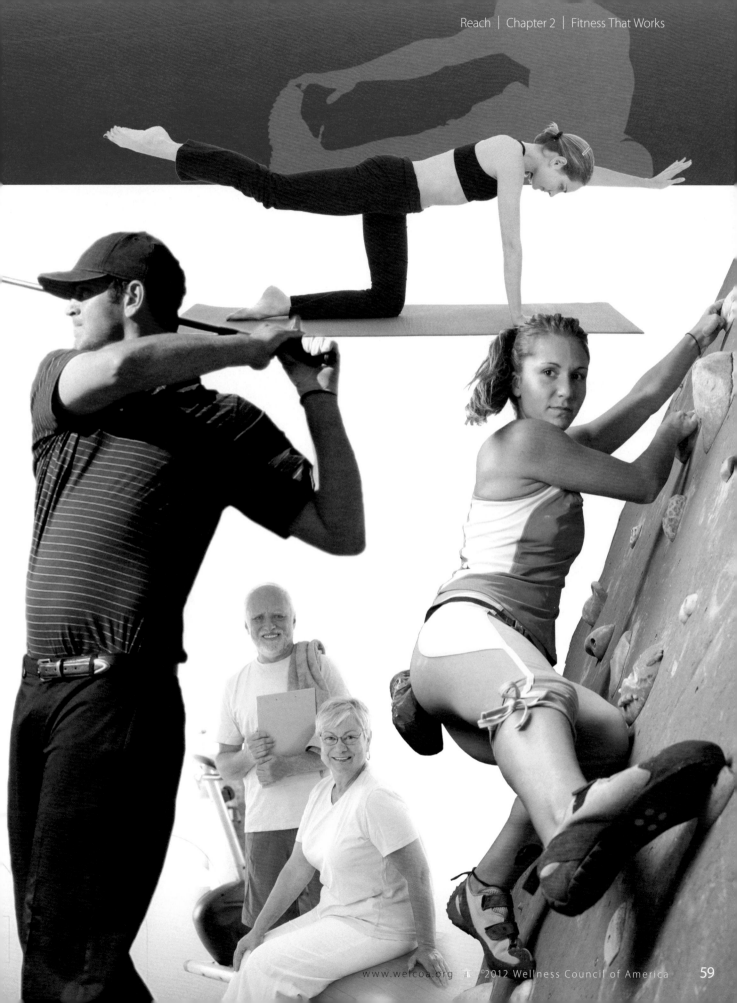

Step

"That's one small step for man, one giant leap for mankind."

—Neil Armstrong

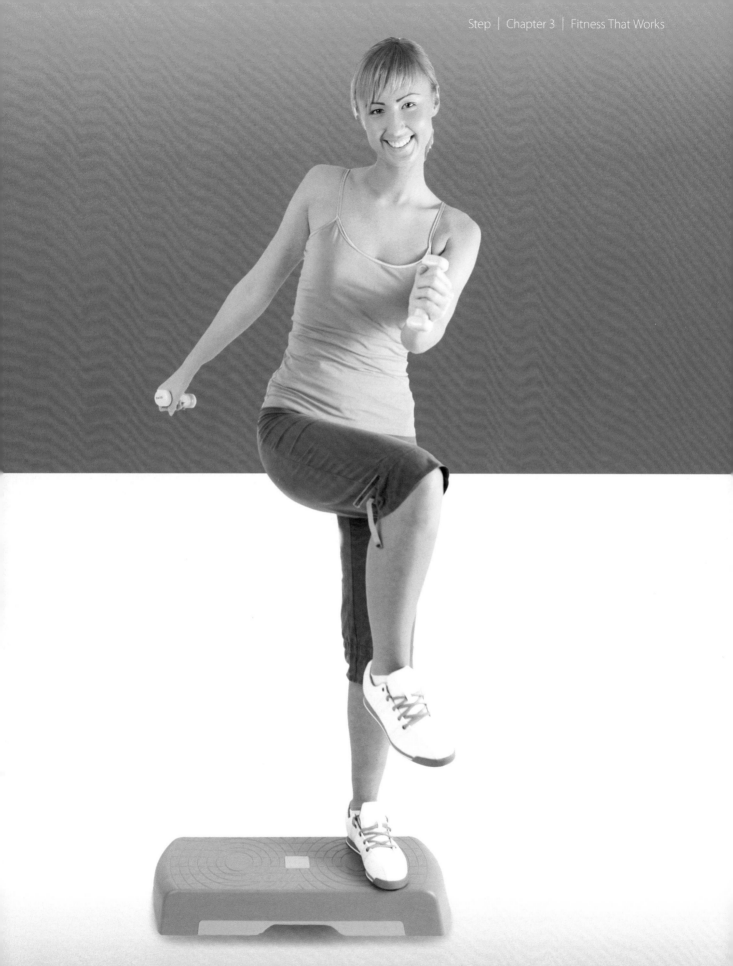

Step

HAVEN'T WE ALL HEARD THOSE FAMOUS WORDS FROM THE JUBILANT AMERICAN ASTRONAUT, NEIL ARMSTRONG, WHEN HE TOOK THIS HISTORIC, FIRST STEP ON THE MOON'S ROCKY SURFACE?

Have you ever wondered what it would have been like to be Neil Armstrong on that momentous day? What would it have felt like to accomplish a dream that, at the time, most of the world thought was impossible? While millions cheered on July 21, 1969 as he made his dramatic descent from the Apollo 11 Lunar Module, most of us had no idea how many other steps it took to get there. Consider the detailed logistical, engineering, mechanical, electrical, aeronautical and physical training steps Neil Armstrong and the entire NASA team had to perform prior to this infamous day.

In this chapter, I want to challenge you to embark upon your own "mission" to take your fitness to another level by taking something as simple, but as ultimately momentous, as a single step. In this chapter, we will look at our third simple move, "step" and how by performing it on a regular basis—just one step at a time—you too can make a giant leap towards your best fitness and health!

We will explore:

1 What is "step?"

2 Why step is so important

3 How inactivity and aging impacts your step

4 How to test your step

5 Simple moves you can do to improve your step

6 Recommended step programs, tools and much more

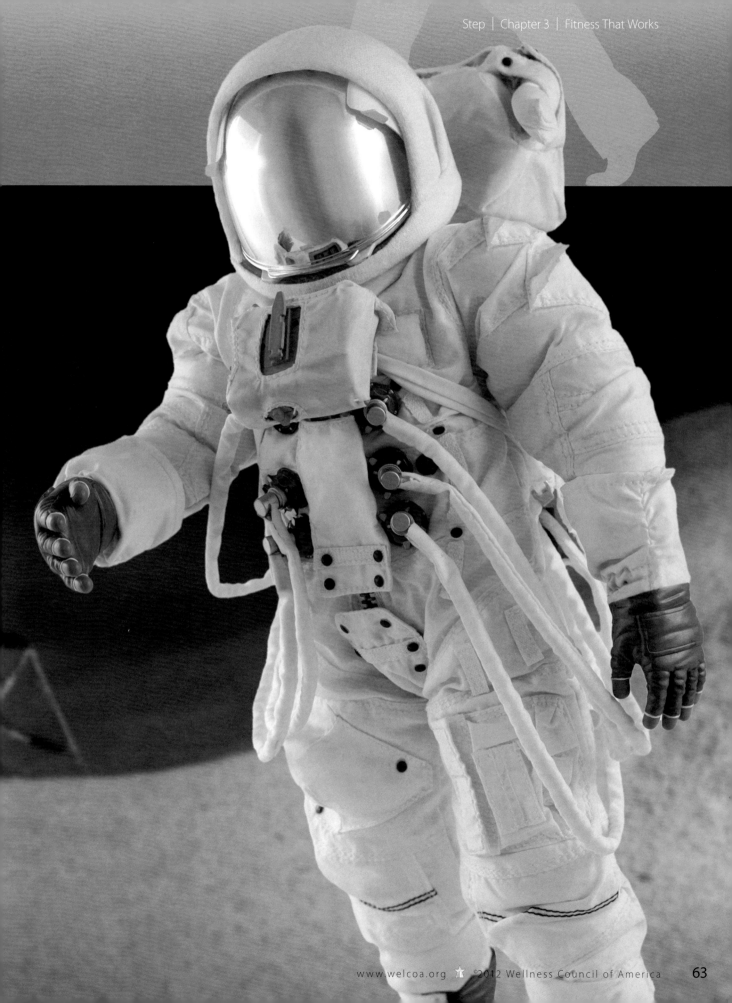

Step

Your First Step!

I had a client named Julie who called me and shared how much she desperately wanted to lose weight and get in shape. Unfortunately, after years of broken diet and exercise promises, she found herself losing the battle. Day after day, Julie just couldn't find the time or energy for exercise. She shared that the simple task of wrestling with the alarm clock and the mounting pressures at work were two of many things that left her defeated and discouraged.

So I asked her to take on a simple assignment. I asked her to describe on a note card (what I call a "Fit Card") that could be placed on her alarm clock at home or computer at work, what her life would be like if she were to decide, each day, to nurture her health and fitness by taking a step. How would going for a short walk in the morning or at break time at work or walking up and down the stairs (instead of taking the elevator at work) look and feel in her life? I asked her to list what potential personal benefits she would experience after four weeks; three months; and one year, if she were to begin to take this small physical daily step. Julie shared after thinking for a moment, "Oh, I would feel so much better about myself. I would be healthier. I'd finally knock my blood pressure and cholesterol down—which have been off the charts for a long, long time. I'd probably improve my stress levels and energy during the workday too. And I know I would lose weight, and finally be able to fit into my "skinny jeans" and all the beautiful work clothes I haven't been able to pull up or button up for a years! I also would probably be more productive in my job, and my kids and co-workers would probably see me in a better mood." She went on and on for at least five minutes, describing all the benefits she would experience by taking a step. Writing each point and pausing occasionally to tell me about it while waving her hands in the air, she became so excited, then smiled and tilted her head to the side, dreaming of "what life could be like."

Then I asked her—when she appeared to be finished sharing—to read this Fit Card at least three times during the day, especially in the morning when the alarm clock went off and during morning, lunch or afternoon work breaks.

She looked at me a little funny. "That's it?" she asked. "That's it!" I said. "You don't want me to exercise?" she retorted. I told her, "If you'd

TAKE YOUR FIRST STEP!

Think about taking your first step by creating your own Fit Card. Describe on a note card that you can carry with you daily (or post on your alarm clock or computer at work) what your health, fitness and life will be like if you were to decide each day to nurture your health and fitness by taking a step (such as walking, jogging, stair climbing, etc.) on a regular basis.

1. List what potential personal benefits you will experience four weeks, three months and one year from today if you were to begin to step regularly.

2. List how you would feel about yourself if you were to step on a regular basis.

3. List the positive benefits that your family, friends and co-workers would experience by you taking a step on a regular basis.

4. On the other side of your card, list the potential challenges you would contend with by taking a step on a regular basis. Write down a potential solution next to each challenge.

I would encourage you to write your answers down on a note card that you can carry with you, or post it where you can read it daily.

Like Julie, commit to follow this simple step and watch what happens!

like, go ahead, but what I really want you to do is read all the benefits you'll experience in your life if you were to take a step and exercise." She smiled and let out a sigh of relief. I then asked her how confident she felt in reading her Fit Card at least three times during the day. She stated, "Oh, I am almost 100% confident that I can do that."

After four weeks Julie contacted me and was excited to share that something amazing had happened!

She mentioned, "The first few days, I found myself hitting the snooze button on the alarm clock as usual. But, the difference was I couldn't go back to sleep without feeling a strong pull to get up and read my card." Regarding work, she mentioned, "At first, I would just ignore reading my Fit Card, but it would beckon me throughout the day and I found it difficult to avoid. After the third day, when the alarm went off, I'd wake right up and think about my card. I began to read it in detail. I'd lie there thinking about getting up and going for a walk and dreamt of how good I'd feel and look if I did it."

She said, "Sean, after two more days of reading my Fit Card in the morning as well as at work, I finally found myself really wanting to go for a walk. I was waking up thinking about how good I would feel and how much more energy I would have." Then she said, "Sean, I did it! I actually woke up and went for a walk every day for an entire week. I even took the stairs during my break times and it felt fantastic! I was so proud of myself." She said, "Now, I don't even have to read my Fit Card anymore because I automatically think about how good I'll feel, how my family, friends and co-workers benefit by me taking time for me. I know if I ever do wrestle with feeling like I want to stay in bed or keep working without a break, I'll just pull out my trusty Fit Card and think about how much better I'll feel!"

The most encouraging news about Julie is she is an avid walker today (she even takes the stairs at work during her morning and afternoon breaks) and has gotten a host of co-workers to join along with her. It was easy for others to follow Julie's path, especially after they saw her amazing transformation. She lost over 50 pounds and lowered her cholesterol and blood pressure to a healthy level. Julie is now fit, trim, healthy and happy. And best of all, in Julie's opinion, she had to buy a number of new clothes and some new jeans. Even her old "skinny jeans" were just way too big!

Step

What Is Step?

The dictionary defines "step" as any movement made by the lifting of your foot and setting it back down again in a new position (either further forward, backwards, up, down or to the side, along with a shifting of your weight in the direction of the new position). Bottom line, we use step in almost any physical activity requiring us to move, including activities and exercises such as: walking, hiking, jogging or stair climbing, just to name a few. But, if you think about all the other various "non-exercise" activities and movements you perform throughout your day that require you to take a step, you'll be thrilled to learn how simple it will be for you to make great strides to improve your fitness and health—even from 9 to 5.

The Goal Of Step And Why It Is So Important

The goal of step is simple: to increase and improve your cardiovascular endurance (as well as strengthen your respiratory system) and reduce the risk of a number of diseases (such as heart disease, diabetes and obesity). Step is a form of activity also known as cardiovascular or aerobic exercise, which, according to Stanford University Medical School researchers, "is any activity that is continuous in movement involving the large muscle groups for an extended period of time, conditioning your heart and lungs by increasing oxygen intake." So, step (like other aerobic or cardiovascular exercises) helps your heart, lungs and body stay fit and young, empowering you to keep moving for a long, long time. The good news is that since your heart is a muscle—you can strengthen it, just like any other muscle.

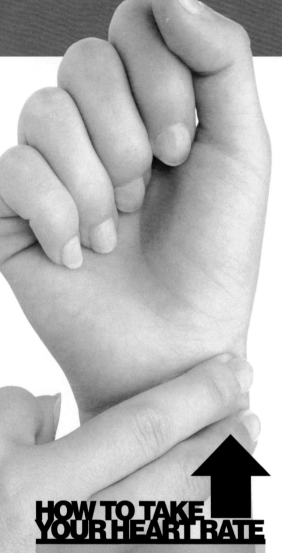

HOW TO TAKE YOUR HEART RATE

Place your index and middle finger gently on the lateral (or thumb) side of the base of your wrist, and feel for your radial artery to check your pulse. Press very gently and you'll feel a beating sensation. This is your heart rate or pulse rate. Next, count how many beats you feel in a 15 second time period. Then multiply your score by four. For example, if you counted 20 beats in 15 seconds, multiply 20 × 4 = a heart rate of 80 beats per minute.

BRAIN TRAIN

What is one of the most powerful muscles in the human body?

The heart.

We so frequently take the heart for granted. This incredible muscle is responsible for all "steps" you take and all human movement. Taking the stairs at work, walking your dog, moving from your kitchen to the living room, strolling through a park or walking on the beach are all activities you can perform because of a healthy heart muscle. Did you know that the heart sends blood in amounts equal to 1,400 gallons a day—or roughly 37 million gallons over a 72-year lifetime—through vessels called arteries which carry necessary oxygen to working muscles? Best of all, it does all this by itself, without any thought or action on our part. Not to mention, the heart delivers oxygen to our brain, which must receive oxygen just to function. Without the heart, we would not be able to breathe, smell, hear, talk, feel, think or survive. Everything from your toes to your brain is dependent upon this fist-sized dynamo!

I often refer to this muscle as a "SMART Muscle" because it performs countless important functions all by itself. For example, the heart muscle has the ability to maintain its own rhythm, beating some 80 times per minute without even thinking about it. This marvelous "energizer bunny" keeps going and going 24/7. Beating about 100,800 times per day, and 36.8 million times a year. Now that's a SMART muscle!

I remember when my son, Joel, was diagnosed with a heart arrhythmia at the age of three. Believe me when I say that my wife and I appreciated every little beat from our little guy's heart. We would spend countless days and nights putting our hands on his little chest to see how he was doing.

To appreciate this magnificent muscle, I'd encourage you tonight to do the same. Put your hand on your heart and be thankful for its every beat. And remember, performing the simple move of "step" will make this muscle stronger, more efficient and even more powerful.

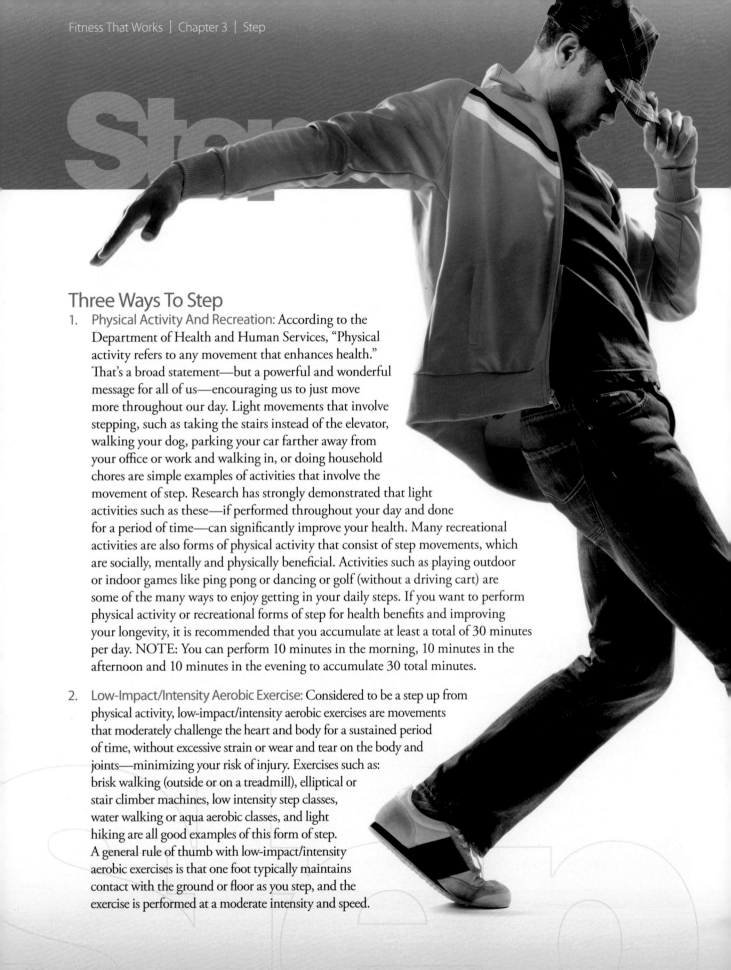

Three Ways To Step

1. Physical Activity And Recreation: According to the Department of Health and Human Services, "Physical activity refers to any movement that enhances health." That's a broad statement—but a powerful and wonderful message for all of us—encouraging us to just move more throughout our day. Light movements that involve stepping, such as taking the stairs instead of the elevator, walking your dog, parking your car farther away from your office or work and walking in, or doing household chores are simple examples of activities that involve the movement of step. Research has strongly demonstrated that light activities such as these—if performed throughout your day and done for a period of time—can significantly improve your health. Many recreational activities are also forms of physical activity that consist of step movements, which are socially, mentally and physically beneficial. Activities such as playing outdoor or indoor games like ping pong or dancing or golf (without a driving cart) are some of the many ways to enjoy getting in your daily steps. If you want to perform physical activity or recreational forms of step for health benefits and improving your longevity, it is recommended that you accumulate at least a total of 30 minutes per day. NOTE: You can perform 10 minutes in the morning, 10 minutes in the afternoon and 10 minutes in the evening to accumulate 30 total minutes.

2. Low-Impact/Intensity Aerobic Exercise: Considered to be a step up from physical activity, low-impact/intensity aerobic exercises are movements that moderately challenge the heart and body for a sustained period of time, without excessive strain or wear and tear on the body and joints—minimizing your risk of injury. Exercises such as: brisk walking (outside or on a treadmill), elliptical or stair climber machines, low intensity step classes, water walking or aqua aerobic classes, and light hiking are all good examples of this form of step. A general rule of thumb with low-impact/intensity aerobic exercises is that one foot typically maintains contact with the ground or floor as you step, and the exercise is performed at a moderate intensity and speed.

> *Research has strongly demonstrated that light activities such as these—if performed throughout your day and done for a period of time—can significantly improve your health.*

3. High-Impact/Intensity Aerobic Exercise: Stepping up to a higher level of intensity and rigor, high-impact/intensity aerobic exercises are movements that significantly challenge the heart and body for a sustained period of time, with greater demands upon the heart, lungs, muscles and joints. Movements such as: running, sprinting, stair running, interval training, wrestling, martial arts and competitive basketball are all examples of this more challenging form of step. A general rule of thumb is that high-impact/intensity aerobic exercises typically require both feet to lose contact with the ground or floor, and are higher in intensity and/or speed.

For low-impact or high-impact step activities, it is recommended that you perform these movements anywhere from 20–60 minutes in duration. This is the length of time required for most aerobic exercises to help improve cardiovascular and overall fitness and health. The higher the intensity of the movement, the lower the duration can be. If you are typically pressed for time and would like to significantly improve your fitness, increase metabolic rate and burn fat more efficiently, turn to page 76 to learn more about interval training.

Remember, regardless of the type of step you choose, always warm up properly.

Benefits: All of the above forms of step have overwhelming scientific evidence to support the growing number of positive benefits for your body and health, including:

- Reduced risk of heart disease, cancer, diabetes, high cholesterol and osteoporosis;
- Strengthened immune system;
- Lower levels of depression, stress and anxiety;
- Increased self-esteem and self-image;
- Improved quality of life;
- Better management of body weight;
- Increased ability to burn fat for energy;
- Better sleep and more energy;
- Stronger bones;
- Increased productivity and improved creativity;
- And the list goes on and on.

Step

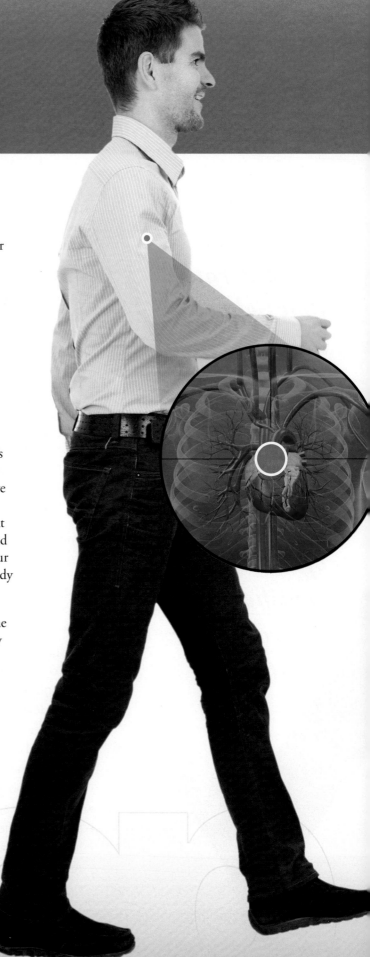

How Inactivity And Aging Impacts Your Step

Picture yourself walking up a flight of stairs. How do you feel? No problem, right? OK, now let's take another flight, and then another, and another and another. Now, how do you feel? No problem? Slightly winded? Moderately winded? Fatigued? Breathless? Your ability to step up three, four or even five flights of stairs is strongly dependent upon the condition, strength and age of your heart. Unfortunately, as we grow older, just past the age of 30, a number of gradual changes begin to occur to our bodies—specifically to our heart and cardiovascular system—that make walking up any flight of stairs exceedingly more difficult. Research demonstrates that as we age, our heart becomes smaller, weaker and less efficient. This affects the heart's ability to pump blood, and transport oxygen and other necessary nutrients to awaiting tissues that help us move our body and get up those darn stairs. Combined with a number of other age-related challenges, such as weight gain, the thickening of the blood and the narrowing and hardening of the arteries due to stored fatty deposits, our heart is left to work considerably harder, leaving our body breathless and searching for an elevator.

The bad news is that we can't stop the "tick-tock" of the aging clock. The good news is that we can significantly slow it down—and get up those stairs! As scientific research clearly demonstrates, many of the challenges and health issues related to aging can be thwarted and delayed by taking a step. For example, a landmark study appearing in the prestigious *Journal of the American Medical Association* (JAMA), uncovered the benefits of performing simple and low impact stepping motions, such as walking up and down a corridor on a consistent basis. The study found these stepping motions considerably lowered the risk of disease, disability and significantly increase mobility and mortality of elderly subjects.

> ## "We do not stop exercising because we grow old—we grow old because we stop exercising."
>
> — **Dr. Kenneth Cooper**
> "The Father of Aerobics,"
> Cooper Institute

If taking small steps such as walking up and down a corridor over a period of time can benefit individuals in their later years of life, just think of what performing a variety of stepping motions at work can do for your body and life. To help you reach your very best in fitness and health, let's take a look at some moves you can do to improve your step.

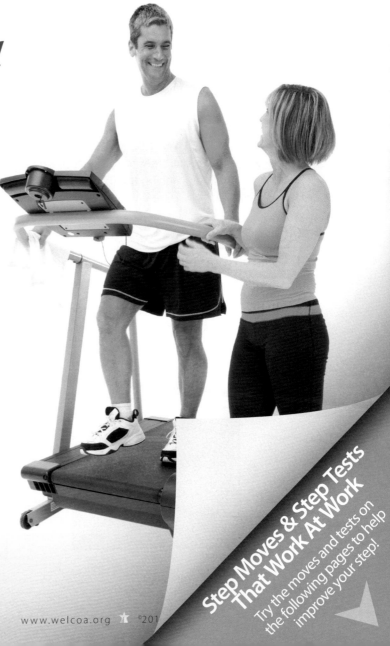

Step Moves & Step Tests That Work At Work

Try the moves and tests on the following pages to help improve your step!

It's time to improve your…
Step

It's time to move…

Step Move #1: Stair Stepping

When at work, one of the best and most convenient ways to challenge your cardiovascular system and keep your heart, lungs and body in shape is to walk up and down stairs.

➤ GET READY

All you'll need is a flight or more of stairs (If you don't have access to stairs, you can also use a low to moderate-sized bench, sturdy chair, outside curb or even a hard-covered, large book placed securely against a wall).

➤ GET SET

Stand upright with your feet together, legs straight and hands down by your sides—facing the lowest step.

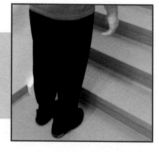

➤ GO

1. Step up with your right foot. Then step up with your left foot.

2. Continue this progression all the way up the flight of stairs.

3. Repeat this motion up and down the stairs with the goal of stepping up and down for at least 4-30 minutes in duration.

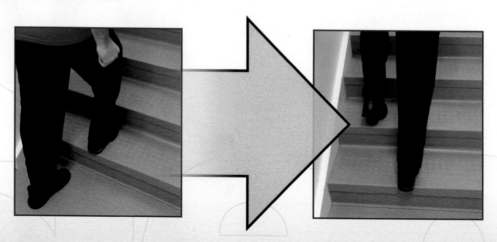

MAINTAIN PROPER FORM

Pointers To Remember:
- ✓ Be sure to properly warm your body up before stair-stepping
- ✓ Keep your back straight while slightly leaning forward from the hips
- ✓ Glance at stairs from time to time
- ✓ Place entire foot on the stairs and press up from the ball and not heel of foot

Common Mistakes To Avoid:
- ✓ Performing stairs too quickly with no warm up
- ✓ Leaning too far forward when climbing stairs
- ✓ Locking knees as you walk up stairs
- ✓ Descending too quickly
- ✓ Pulling self up with hand rail

VARIATIONS

Beginners:
- ✓ Walk up stairs slowly
- ✓ Lightly place hand onto stair railing for extra support
- ✓ Rest before preceding up next flight of stairs
- ✓ Use a small step, curb or book to practice the stepping movement if too difficult

Intermediate/Advanced:
- ✓ Take two steps at a time (great for strengthening buttocks and thighs)
- ✓ Walk up the stairs sideways (great way to work inner and outer thighs)
- ✓ Pump your arms quickly
- ✓ Jog up and walk down stairs
- ✓ Sprint up and jog down stairs

FAQ

How often should I perform Simple Step Moves That Work? You can perform step moves daily, every day of the week, but for best results, I recommend cross training or performing different types of "steps" on varying days of the week (e.g. stair walking on Monday, stair jogging on Tuesday, stair walking on Wednesday, stair running/sprinting on Thursday, stair walking by taking two steps at a time on Friday, etc.)

Note: Depending upon your personality, see what works best for you—but the more you can practice step moves, the better.

How long should I perform Simple Step Moves That Work? To answer this question, it depends upon your goals, time restrictions and type of step chosen. But, if you are planning to perform the Simple Step Moves at work, it is recommended you perform stair-stepping anywhere from 4-30 minutes per day. (Remember, you can break up your stair stepping throughout your day, by taking the stairs in the morning, afternoon and before leaving work.) Also, if you'd like, instead of tracking time you can set a goal of "counting" the number of steps you accumulate throughout your day by using a simple device called a pedometer.

How difficult should the Simple Step Moves That Work be? Based upon your fitness level, you should begin at a level that is comfortable, but also challenging for you. You can progress from beginning to more challenging levels as you improve. You can take the step test to track your progress and set goals. Regarding your goals and intensity with step, here are some things to consider.

According to Dr. Kenneth Cooper and The Cooper Institute: If you are interested in improving longevity and health, perform physical activity or recreational activity at any pace, regardless of heart rate response.

To improve your aerobic fitness and or manage your weight, challenge your body by increasing your heart rate. When stepping, you should be challenged to carry on a long and lengthy conversation, but should be able to talk in short three word sentences. If you can't converse at all, you are going too fast. If you can sing comfortably, you are going too slowly. Another way of measuring your heart rate is using a heart rate monitor .

Note: To determine a rough estimate of your maximum heart rate, subtract your current age from the number 220 if you are male and 226 if you are female (e.g. 220 – Age = Maximum Heart Rate for a male). You can either increase or decrease your stair-stepping intensity by looking at the variations of the simple moves on this page.

It's time to test your...
Step

Now, let's take a moment to identify how well you step. By performing the simple step test, you'll be able to determine how strong your heart, lungs and muscles are.

Step Test #1: Stair Stepping

Having a strong heart and lungs (cardiovascular and respiratory systems) are two of the most important aspects related to your physical fitness and an active, energetic life. Stepping is one of the best ways you can test how strong your heart and lungs are, measuring your cardiovascular endurance and stamina.

➤ GET READY

You'll need a 12 inch bench or step (note: You can use the bottom step of a flight of stairs at work or home), a flat non-slip flooring on which to step up and down, a stop watch, clock or wrist watch with a second hand to time yourself, a pencil or pen, and this book to score your results.

➤ GET SET

Stand upright with your feet together, legs straight and hands down by your sides—facing the step.

➤ GO

1. Start the clock when you step up with your right foot. Then step up with your left foot. Then step down with your right foot and down with your left foot. Moving in a cadence of "Up, Up, Down, Down," try to maintain this steady pace for three minutes. (If you are interested, this would be a cadence of 96 beats per minute. If you have access to a metronome, you can set it to 96 beats per minute and follow the rhythm of the metronome for your stepping. If not, say out loud, "Up, Up, Down, Down, Up, Up, Down, Down," etc. in a steady rhythm—moving in-step with your verbal cues for three minutes.

2. At the end of three minutes, stop, remain standing and immediately check your heart rate by taking your pulse for one minute. Then write it down. (For more information, see the sidebar on page 67: "How To Take Your Heart Rate").

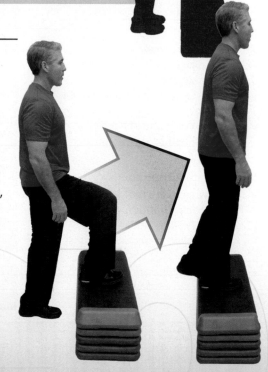

YOUR SCORE

See how you did by comparing your scores with the scores below. Find your age, gender and your estimated score in the following scale. Circle how you scored.

MALE	18-25	26-35	36-45	46-55	56-65	65+
Excellent Scores	<79	<81	<83	<87	<86	<88
Average Scores	100-105	100-107	104-112	106-116	104-112	104-113

FEMALE	18-25	26-35	36-45	46-55	56-65	65+
Excellent Scores	<85	<88	<90	<94	<95	<90
Average Scores	109-117	112-119	111-118	116-120	113-118	116-122

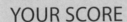

COUNT YOUR STEPS

A handy little device that I find very helpful in motivating my clients to step is a pedometer—a matchbox-sized gadget that clips onto a belt, pants, or skirt waist and records the number of steps taken each day. When beginning your "Fitness That Works" program, I recommend using a pedometer with the following step goals in mind:

✓ For the Beginning Stepper: 5,000 total steps a day is an achievable, but challenging first goal;

✓ For the Medium-Stepper, 10,000 steps a day;

✓ For the "I Love To Step" individual, try to accumulate 20,000 steps a day.

✓ Track your average number of steps each day, week and month; and

✓ At the end of four weeks, average your number of steps per month.

No matter what level of Stepper you are, each day (or as a weekly average), plot the number of steps you take on a chart that you can view daily. Plotting your steps helps you visualize your progress. To determine your fitness level and assess your progress, be sure and perform the Step Test on the previous page every four to six weeks.

Fitness That Works Challenge: Regardless of the type of step chosen or your fitness level, make it a goal to go up and down at least one flight of stairs every day. Who knows? Pretty soon your heart will be so strong you'll be able to reach the moon.

Step

Since there are a few different ways to improve your step, what should I be mindful of?

To improve your step, you can perform simple movements such as those mentioned on page 72-73. Or you can select from various recommended programs and tools based upon your Fitness That Works Personality Profile. **Note:** All programs, tools or activities that are checked are recommended for you.

Fitness Personality Profile—My Personality Profile Is

▼ Check three that are the most appealing to you.

STEP ACTIVITIES/EXERCISES	PROFILE A	PROFILE B	PROFILE C
☐ Simple Moves - Stair Stepping (See page 72–73)	✓	✓	✓
☐ Physical Activity (e.g. Walking the dog, parking your car farther away from your office or work and walking in, household chores such as vacuuming, mopping and gardening)	✓		✓
☐ Light Walking (Outside)	✓		✓
☐ Recreational Sports (e.g. Softball, Golf, Ping Pong, Tennis, Racquetball)		✓	✓
☐ Dancing (e.g. Line Dancing, Ballet, Hip Hop, Modern, Swing, Flamenco and Latin)		✓	
☐ Skating (Ice or In Line)			✓
☐ Stair Master Machine (Stair Stepping)	✓		
☐ Step Ups	✓		
☐ Power Walking (On a treadmill/street)	✓		✓
☐ Jogging (On a treadmill/street)	✓		✓
☐ Elliptical Machine	✓		
☐ Hiking	✓		✓
☐ Cross Country Skiing	✓		✓
☐ Snow Shoeing	✓		✓
☐ Beach Walking/Running	✓		
☐ Brisk Beach Walking/Running	✓		✓
☐ Water Aerobics Classes		✓	
☐ Trampoline Stepping	✓		✓
☐ Martial Arts (e.g. Aikido, Judo, Jujutsu, Kendo, Karate, Kung Fu, Mixed Martial Arts, Jeet Kune Do, Taekwondo)	✓	✓	
☐ Rock Climbing	✓		✓
☐ Aerobics Classes (e.g. Step, Jazzercise, Zumba, Boot Camp, Gliding, Cardio Kick-boxing, Tae Boe, Stroller-Fit)		✓	
☐ Cardio DVD Workouts (e.g. Walking, Dancing, Step, Interval Training)	✓		
☐ Rope Jumping	✓		
☐ Counting Steps With A Pedometer (See page 75)	✓		✓
☐ Interval Training (Stair Stepping/Walking, Walking/Jogging, Sprinting/Jogging, Track Sprinting/Running, Jumping Rope)	✓		
☐ Competitive Sports (Basketball, Soccer, Lacrosse, Hockey, Wrestling, or Tackle, Touch or Flag Football)		✓	✓
☐ 10 Minute 4–3–2–1 Fitness Training (See pages 148–149)	✓	✓	✓

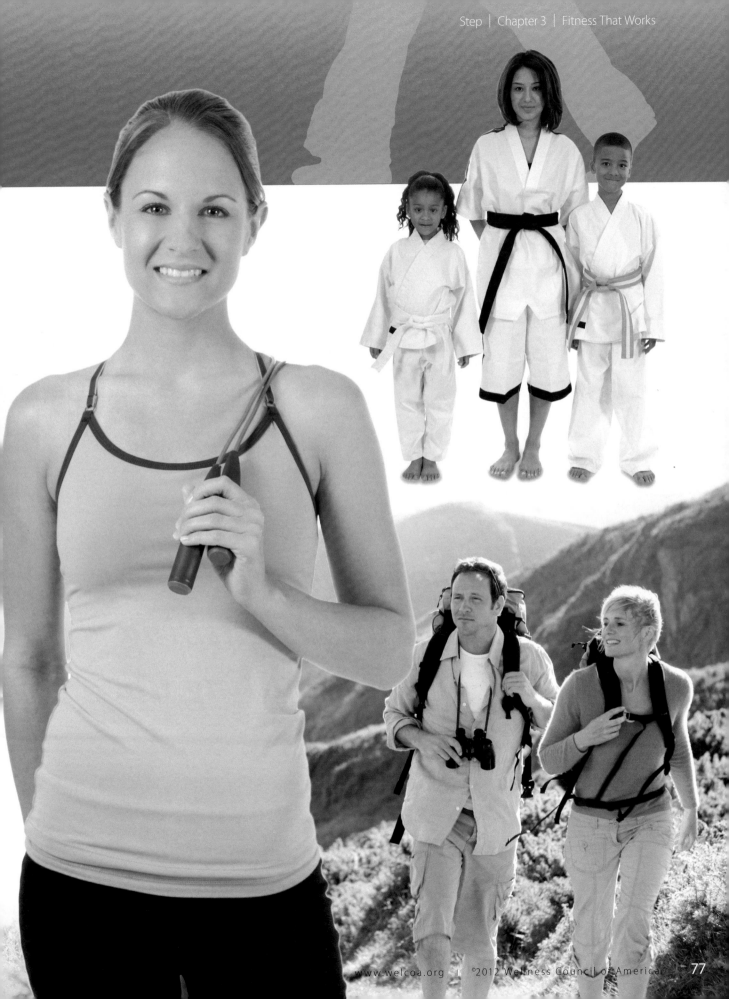

Push & Pull

"*There are two ways of exerting one's strength: one is pushing down, the other is pulling up.*"

—Booker T. Washington

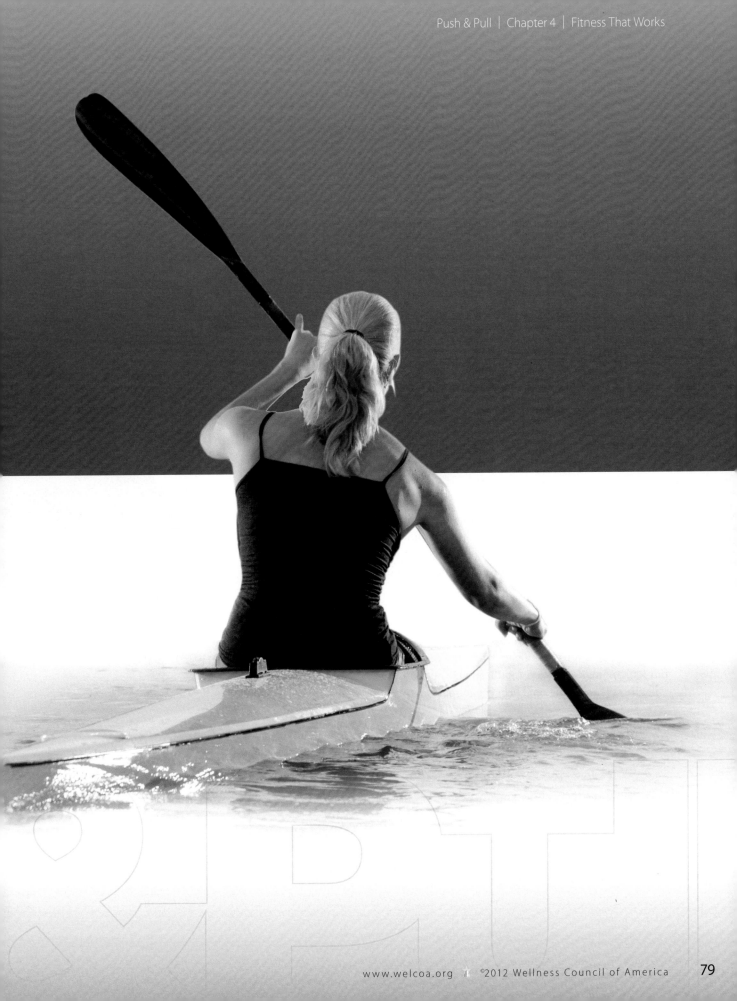

Push&Pull

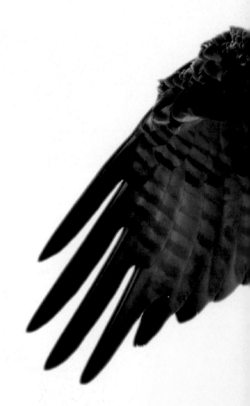

NESTLED IN THE WARMTH OF HER MOTHER'S WINGS AND PERCHED HIGH UPON A BLACK, JAGGED PINNACLE, A BABY EAGLET SOON WILL EMBARK UPON A FEAT ONLY FAMILIAR IN HER DREAMS. Over the centuries, young eaglets have learned to fly (and ultimately soar) through an ancient ritual: they are "pushed" by their guardian out of their secure, fortified nests. What is not commonly shared about this beautiful rite of passage are the days of deprivation from food that "Mama" and "Papa" initiate to gently "pull" their young one out of her comfort zone. All is planned to coerce their fledgling to follow their lead. After countless days of malnutrition, "Mama Eagle" suddenly and abruptly leaves the nest and captures dinner. She then heads back to the nest with the long-awaited feast in her claws, and flies by ever so closely to draw her baby's attention. Making repeated fly-bys in an attempt to entice her hungry young to follow, "Mama" uses a balance of "pushing" and "pulling" over and over again until finally, her baby bravely leaps to follow— taking "Mama's" lead (and dinner!).

When we think about any success we may have experienced in our lives, we also had to participate in a similar dance of "push" and "pull." If you talk to any successful person who has accomplished a significant goal in their life, you'll usually hear about someone else who encouraged, motivated, coached, and "pushed and/or pulled" them—beyond their limitations or what they thought possible—to reach their dreams.

In this chapter, I want you to think of me as another coach, friend, or "Papa Eagle," ready to challenge you to leap to greater heights with your fitness and health. While I won't be enticing you with "dinner," I will be showing you our fourth simple move, push-pull, and how performing it on a regular basis will give you new wings and help you to soar.

We will explore:

1 What is push-pull?

2 Why is push-pull so important?

3 How inactivity and aging impacts your push-pull

4 Simple moves you can do to improve your push-pull

5 How to test your push-pull

6 Recommended push-pull programs, tools and much more

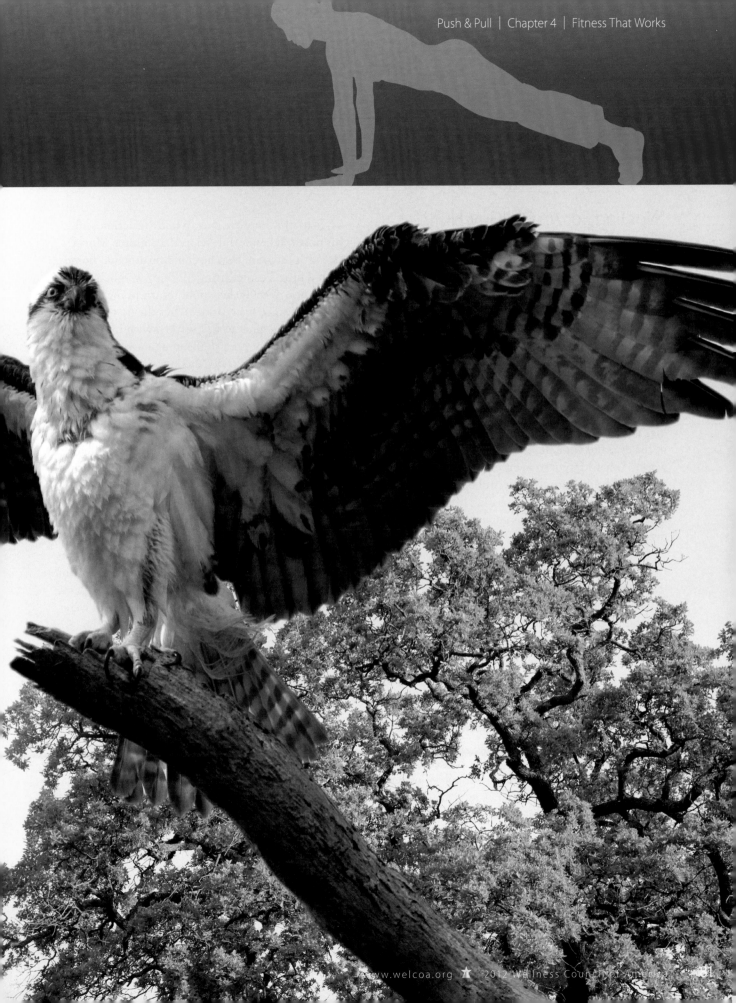

Push & Pull

"Not Bad For An Old Guy, Huh?"

I'll never forget the day I met Byron. I was sitting in a chair in a private fitness center, taking a break while waiting for my new training client to arrive. Suddenly, he entered the doorway. Walking in—or should I say, shuffling in—he entered the room and came directly towards me. With thick-rimmed black glasses, a red tank top and plaid shorts that were too big for his thin body, he smiled and slowly extended his hand as he said, "Pleasure to meet you, Sean! Are you ready to train the next State Power Lifting Champion?" I politely smiled and shook his hand. Then, he lowered his eye glasses, rose up on his toes, looked me square in the eye, and with all seriousness said, "Let's get to work!" What I forgot to mention is that Byron was a 68 year old, 146 pound, successful business executive from a local corporation who hadn't lifted a weight in 20 some years—but as I was about to find out, he was dead serious!

Initially, I took Byron through a number of fitness tests to determine if he was healthy enough to exercise, as well as identify any particular weaknesses and ascertain his "real" goals (I really didn't think the power lifting idea was legit). One thing I noticed right away with Byron was his lack of upper body strength and postural problems. He mentioned to me that he spent quite a bit of time sitting at work and on airplanes—and that he had neglected his fitness for too long. I asked him to complete a couple of muscular endurance tests using his body weight, including a push-up test and a modified pull-up test. (Both of which he scored in the "poor" category for his age bracket).

To help him improve overall body function and his postural issues, I developed a "Simple Moves" strength program that he could do at work, home or at a fitness center using his body weight and light resistance. Weekly, he would return to me and I would advance his routine. After the first six weeks, he was doing quite well. I worked with him to help him progress to more challenging movements. Then after 12 weeks, we tested again to see how his upper body strength had improved. We were both surprised! His push-up and pull-up scores were excellent! He scored in the "good" category—but get this—for an 18 year old male! Byron cracked a smile and said, "Not bad for an old guy, huh? But, we've still got a long way to go to get to that State Championship!" I hadn't really taken Byron seriously, until that day.

He then asked me to prepare him for his first power lifting competition—which was to be in eight weeks. We went to work on strengthening his body, taking his training to another level. He enjoyed every minute of it—as he was becoming the talk of his company, the fitness center and the community. We all were amazed at the progress he was making and the transformation to his body and his life—he looked years younger, stronger and happier. The day of the event came. I thought if he could just compete and place in the top 20, it would be cause for celebration. Well, there was cause for celebration, when on his first competition Byron came home with the first place trophy! At age 68, he beat out many men half his age in his weight class. Over the following months, Byron continued to diligently train, performing his strength exercises and ultimately, after a number of victorious competitions, he won the State Power Lifting Championship at 68 years old! I'll never forget that day, nor Byron's signature question as he hoisted the trophy high above his head and smiled, "Not bad for an old guy, huh?" Not bad indeed, Byron!

MUSCULAR BALANCE

"Sit Up Straight And Listen"

How's your posture? Do you stand tall and upright? Is your chest up? Are your shoulders "relaxed, strong and back" or "rounded and drawn forward?"

The latest research demonstrates that sitting too much can create muscular imbalances and postural problems. With chest muscles pulling shoulders forward and making upper back muscles weak, this can lead to "rounded shoulders," or what is also known as "corporate syndrome/upper cross syndrome." A chain of such muscular imbalances can lead to poor posture and a myriad of aches and pains, such as headaches, back problems, fatigue and more.

What are some of the best moves to straighten up?

1. **Move around:** We were not created to sit for long periods of time because as we do, muscles become weaker, tighter and shorter. So, every hour stand up and take a few minutes to move your body—stretch your neck, shoulders, chest and back.

2. **Shoulder retractions:** While sitting at your desk or in a chair, pull your shoulder blades together and back, and hold for a count of four to six seconds. Repeat 10 times at least two to three times during the day.

3. **Follow the 30/30 rule:** When sitting, be mindful of your posture. Place a sticky note on your computer, calendar or desk phone to remind you to sit up tall and strong, or better yet, stand up and relax your shoulders for 30 seconds every 30 minutes. Also, sit upright on the end of your chair throughout the day—avoid leaning to one side as this can create lower and upper back problems later.

4. **Perform an equal amount of push-pull exercises:** Strengthening your push and pull muscles on a regular basis helps to prevent an overdependence on one set of muscles, which can create an imbalance and impact your posture. Also, be sure and strengthen your abdominal, hip and lower back muscles as they are very susceptible to injury, fatigue and weakness.

Push & Pull

What Is Push? What Is Pull?

Did you know that every movement your body makes is in some way dependent upon your muscles? As we have discussed in previous chapters, muscles help us balance, reach, step, walk, breathe, jog, run and as we are now going to see, our upper body muscles (specifically our chest, arms, shoulders and upper back) help us push and pull.

Push: The action of push is any pressing movement made to move or propel something away from you.

Pull: The motion of pull is the opposite of push, which is any action drawing an object closer towards you.

If you think about it, we need our push and pull muscles to be strong for many daily and recreational activities. Consider how often you push such as when you're pushing yourself out of bed or out of a chair, or pushing a loaded shopping cart at the grocery store or a lawn mower (not the self-propelled kind, of course), or catching yourself when you may have slipped or fallen to the ground. Pulling is also a necessary movement for daily living. You'll be happy that your upper body muscles are strong when you need to open a door, or grab a box and pull it closer to you, or pull some stubborn weeds, rake some thick leaves, or climb a ladder, or countless other movements throughout your daily life.

The Goal Of Push-Pull

The goal with the move(s) of push-pull is simple—to help strengthen your upper body (chest, shoulders, arms and back) to enhance your daily living, improve your posture and—oh yes, I almost forgot— tone and tighten the back of your arms. (See The Brain Train on page 85.)

BRAIN TRAIN

Research Demonstrates How To Get Rid Of "Jiggly" Arms!

What is the number one area of the body most women want to improve?

While responses may vary, as a personal trainer, I frequently get asked by many female clients, "How can I get rid of my 'jiggly' arms?" And I must not be the only one getting this question.

A recent study performed by the University of Wisconsin/La Crosse Exercise and Health Program set out to find the best exercises to help tone and strengthen the back of the arms (the triceps). Fifteen healthy women aged 20-24 were recruited for the study and asked to perform eight different "triceps exercises" to measure the impact and effectiveness of each on the back of the arm. Electromyographic (EMG) measurements were taken with each exercise and researchers compared the ratings. They discovered that the top two most effective exercises were achieved by using body-weight, and the third best was performed with simple portable equipment.

The Top Three Triceps ("Push") Exercises:

1. Triangle Push-Ups
2. Bench/Chair Dips
3. Kickbacks (These are best performed with dumbbells, but any resistance such as a water bottle would suffice).

The researchers were thrilled to learn that women and men can effectively strengthen and tone their arms even at work or home. Brittany Boehler, one of the lead researchers says, "Many women are concerned they don't have time to get to the gym or they don't have the necessary exercise equipment at home to get fit. But this research essentially eliminates those excuses. I think the take-home message is that if somebody really wants to work their triceps in a short amount of time, they'll get the most bang for the buck from these three exercises."

Along with a healthy diet, regular cardiovascular (step moves) and push-pull training, you can wave goodbye to those "jiggly" arms!

Push&Pull

Two Ways To Improve Your Push-Pull

ISOTONIC STRENGTH TRAINING. The most common form of improving your push-pull and your muscles is technically referred to as "Isotonic Strength Training." This is a fancy way of saying "any movement causing your muscles to shorten and lengthen, and your joints to bend and straighten in a range of motion against a steady resistance, such as a dumbbell, barbell, resistance tube or even your own body weight." Weight training, such as bicep curls with a dumbbell and/or pull-ups with your body weight, is a good example of this type of training.

BENEFITS ➤

- Strengthens your muscles, tendons, ligaments;
- Improves your posture;
- Tones and firms muscles;
- Decreases your risk of injury;
- Boosts metabolism;
- Improves heart health and bone density;
- Reduces stress and anxiety;
- Lowers risks of cancer, blood pressure, diabetes;
- Reduces pre-menstrual symptoms;
- Improves sleep; and
- Much, much, much more.

ISOMETRIC STRENGTH TRAINING. Isometric strength training is a form of training that was made popular by Charles Atlas in the 1920s, used by NASA astronauts and is still a beneficial and practiced form of exercise today. Unlike isotonic training, isometric movements are "static," or performed without moving your joints. You still flex and relax your muscles, but your joints stay in the same position throughout the exercise. An example of a common format for isometric training would be: trying to push an immovable object such as a wall or parked car, or clasping both hands together and pressing together as hard as you can, while holding the contraction (or flexing your muscles) as hard as you can for 6-10 seconds, then relaxing.

BENEFITS ➤ Isometric strength training, like isotonic, also tones, strengthens and improves muscularity as well as your posture, but with additional benefits.

Isometric Training:
- Is easy to perform without the need of any equipment or special machinery;
- Allows you to complete a full workout in a much faster time frame than isotonic training;
- Allows you the ability to maximize muscular contractions without risk to muscles or joint pain;
- Is one of the best forms of strength training for those who are arthritic or rehabilitation of injured individuals; and
- Has many of the same, listed health and fitness benefits as isotonic training.

PLEASE NOTE—Isometric training can be quite mentally and physically challenging—as you are not moving when performing—so it isn't for everyone.

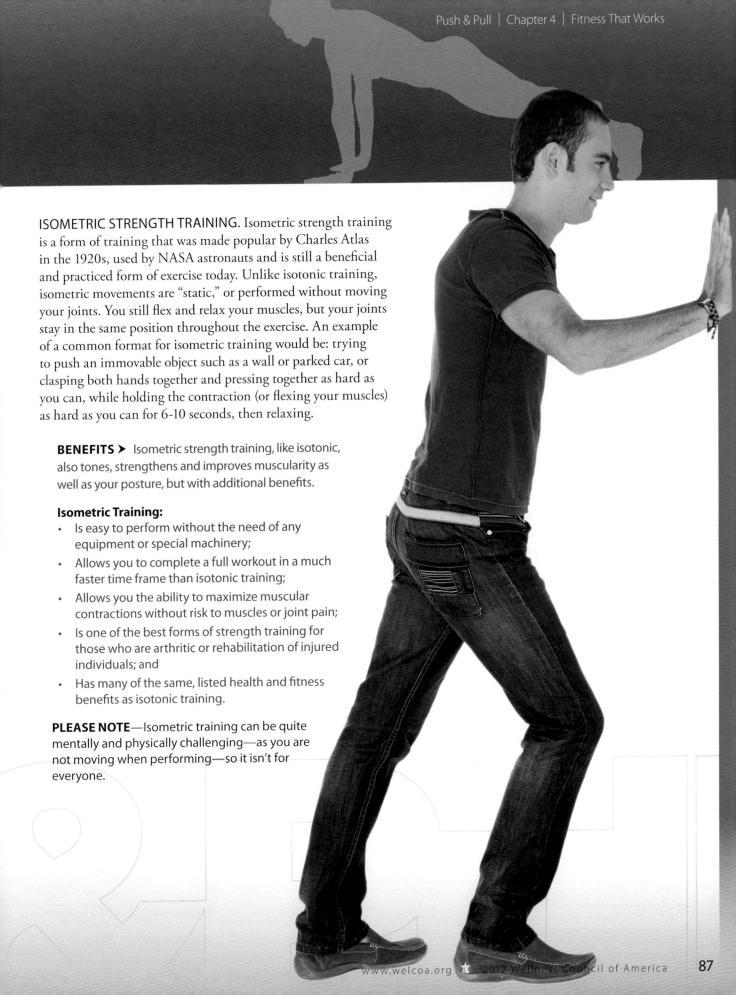

Push&Pull

How Inactivity And Aging Impacts Your Push-Pull

"Do you want to know the secret to life?" snarled "Curly," the wise old cowboy, played by Jack Palance. He was talking to the quiet and meek New York City executive, "Mitch," played by Billy Crystal, in the award-winning movie, "City Slickers." "Curly," raising his hand to hold up his weathered, cowboy index finger, slowly exclaimed, "It's one thing! Once you figure out what your 'one thing' is, everything else is just junk!" While the movie and actors received much acclaim, it was Jack Palance—"Old Curly"—who won the coveted Academy Award for his supporting acting role and performance. At his acceptance speech, the calm, collected and fit 73 year old actor surprised the masses when he dropped to the floor and performed a number of one-arm push-ups with the ease of a 20 year old!

Picture yourself at 70—what do you look like? What do you feel like? How strong are you? How many push-ups do you think you could do on your 70th birthday? Do you think you'll be able to match Jack Palance's one-arm push-up wonders? What was his "one thing"—his secret to staying so fit and strong later in his life?

Researchers and experts in the field of Gerontology (the study of the science of aging) have found as a general rule that our muscle mass (or the size of our muscles) and strength diminish as much as 30% between the ages of 40-70—rapidly decreasing after the age of 45. So, if we do the math—according to the researchers, if you can complete 10 push-ups now at age 40, by age 70 you may only be able to do about two or three—or even less— in your "golden years!" You may be thinking, "Who cares about doing push-ups or other

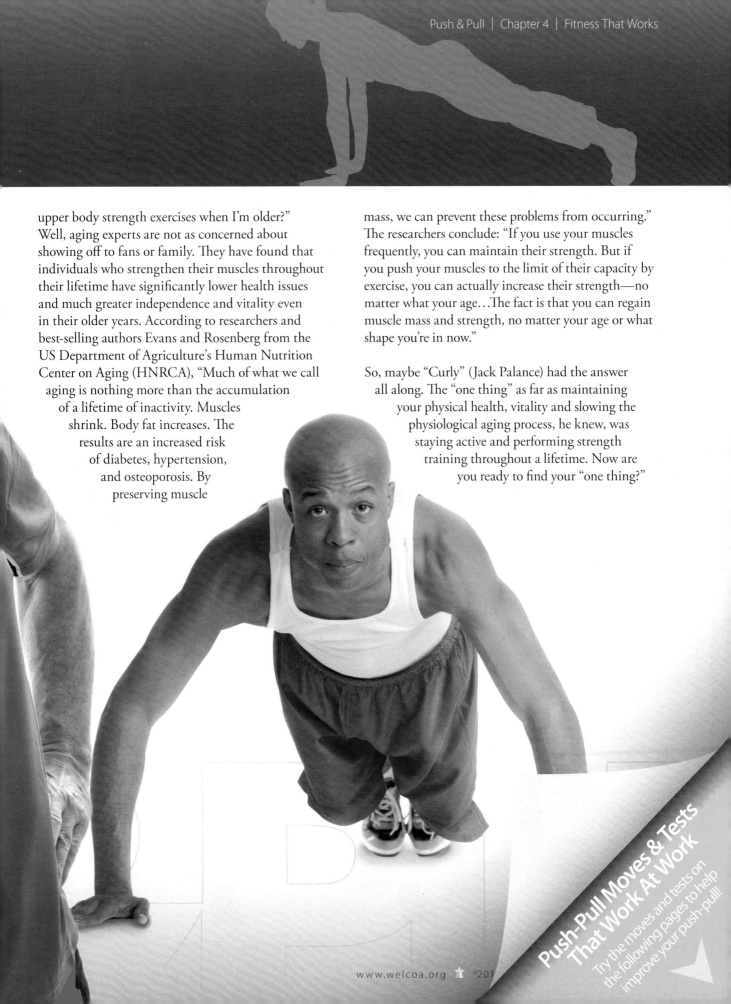

upper body strength exercises when I'm older?" Well, aging experts are not as concerned about showing off to fans or family. They have found that individuals who strengthen their muscles throughout their lifetime have significantly lower health issues and much greater independence and vitality even in their older years. According to researchers and best-selling authors Evans and Rosenberg from the US Department of Agriculture's Human Nutrition Center on Aging (HNRCA), "Much of what we call aging is nothing more than the accumulation of a lifetime of inactivity. Muscles shrink. Body fat increases. The results are an increased risk of diabetes, hypertension, and osteoporosis. By preserving muscle

mass, we can prevent these problems from occurring." The researchers conclude: "If you use your muscles frequently, you can maintain their strength. But if you push your muscles to the limit of their capacity by exercise, you can actually increase their strength—no matter what your age…The fact is that you can regain muscle mass and strength, no matter your age or what shape you're in now."

So, maybe "Curly" (Jack Palance) had the answer all along. The "one thing" as far as maintaining your physical health, vitality and slowing the physiological aging process, he knew, was staying active and performing strength training throughout a lifetime. Now are you ready to find your "one thing?"

Push-Pull Moves & Tests That Work At Work

Try the moves and tests on the following pages to help improve your push-pull!

It's time to improve your…

Push & Pull

It's time to move…

Pull Move #1: Chair Dip

This simple move is one of the most effective exercises to strengthen and tone the back of your arms, chest and shoulders. The best part of this move is you can perform it at work—in your office, manufacturing area, break-room—or even at home.

➤ GET READY

All you'll need is a sturdy chair or bench, and you are on your way!

➤ GET SET

Sit upright on the end of the chair or bench with your knees bent at 90 degrees and feet hip-width apart and feet placed securely on the floor. Also, grasp the end of the chair with palms down and knuckles facing outward. Your hands should be near your thighs, closer than shoulder width apart.

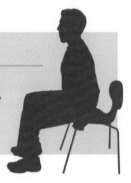

➤ GO

1. Transfer your body weight off the chair by walking your feet out slowly and supporting your weight with your arms extended, maintaining a slight bend in your elbows.

2. Slowly and under control, bend your elbows and allow your body to move down towards the floor—go as far as you comfortably can—elbows to be no more than a 90-degree angle.

3. Straighten your arms, pressing from the heel of both hands, raise your body back to step 1 and repeat 8-12 times or as many as you can safely complete.

NOTE: If you have shoulder, arm, wrist or back problems, we recommend that you not perform this move.

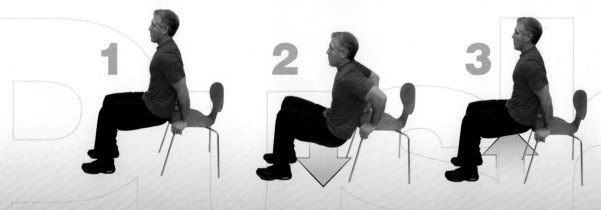

MAINTAIN PROPER FORM

Pointers To Remember:

✓ Eyes looking forward throughout motion
✓ Back straight throughout movement
✓ Go as low as you comfortably can, but no lower than 90 degrees
✓ Elbows slightly bent in upward position
✓ Keep shoulders down throughout motion
✓ Use arms as much as possible and your legs as little as possible

Common Mistakes To Avoid:

✓ Looking down (chin to chest)
✓ Leaning too far forward
✓ Elbows pointing out away from body
✓ Going too low
✓ Locking elbows
✓ Raising shoulders to ears
✓ Pushing too much with legs

VARIATIONS

Beginners:

✓ Stay seated in your chair and press up/down
✓ Keep your feet closer to chair
✓ Place more weight on your legs and less on your arms
✓ Don't go as low in movement

Intermediate/Advanced:

✓ Straighten legs out—weight on heels
✓ Elevate feet on another chair/bench
✓ Add weight in lap (e.g. books, briefcase or weight plates)
✓ Flex triceps muscle in upward position

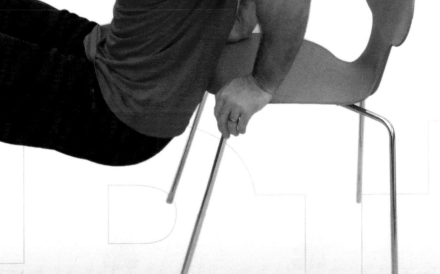

It's time to improve your...
Push & Pull

Now, try this move...

Pull Move #2: Chair Shoulder Retraction Row (With Water Bottles)

To help you improve your posture as well as strengthen your shoulders, arms, upper and lower back, here's a great simple move you can do while seated on a chair or bench at work anytime between 9 to 5.

➤ GET READY

Remember, all you'll need is a chair or bench and a couple of full water bottles, or if you'd like, you can perform this move with one arm at a time using any weighted object, such as a book, briefcase or back pack.

➤ GET SET

Sit upright on the edge of a chair or bench with feet hip-width apart, knees bent and holding two water bottles with arms extended down by your sides.

➤ GO

1. Keeping your head and chest up and eyes looking slightly in front of you, slowly bend forward from the waist, allowing water bottles to hang down by the sides of your thighs, with palms facing in.

2. Next, begin the motion by squeezing your shoulder blades together and bending your elbows, raising the water bottles back and up towards your abdomen/hip area. Remember to keep your arms close to your sides throughout the motion.

3. Lower the water bottles back down and then repeat motion, 8-12 times or as many as you can safely complete.

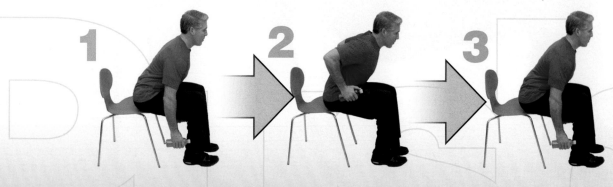

MAINTAIN PROPER FORM

Pointers To Remember:

✓ Initiate the movement by squeezing your shoulder blades together and straight throughout movement
✓ Keep head and chest up throughout movement
✓ Keep abdominal muscles and torso tight throughout motion, allowing only shoulders, upper back and arms to move

Common Mistakes To Avoid:

✓ Pulling with biceps only
✓ Looking down and rounding shoulders
✓ Swinging or rocking lower back or torso to propel weight up towards body
✓ Moving too quickly
✓ Holding breath

VARIATIONS

Beginners:

✓ Perform movement without weight
✓ Place one arm on thighs for support
✓ Move one arm at a time
✓ Perform movement in a chair

Intermediate/Advanced:

✓ Perform movement with heavier resistance (e.g. use a briefcase, purse, medium to large-sized books, and/or dumbbells)
✓ Hold contraction at end point for two to three seconds
✓ Move slower, especially on down motion
✓ Perform movement without a chair

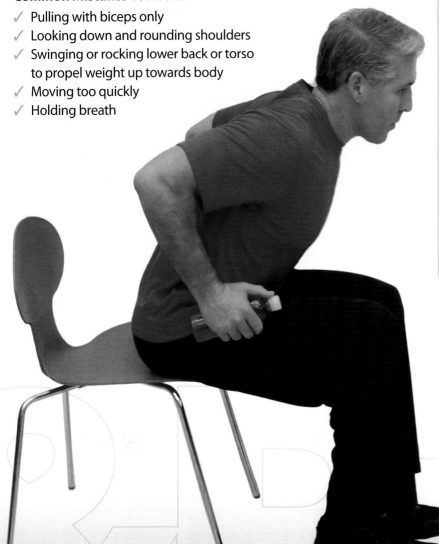

It's time to test your...
Push&Pull

Now, let's take a moment to see how strong your upper body muscles are. Specifically, how strong your push muscles are.

Push-Pull Test #1: Chair Dip Test

Having strong upper body muscles to help you push improves many daily activities. This test measures the muscular endurance of your triceps, chest and shoulders.

➤ GET READY

You'll need a stable, non-moving chair or bench with a hard seat placed on a non-slip surface (preferably positioned against a wall) to sit on, as well as a pencil or pen and this book to score your results.

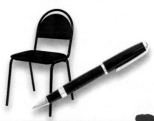

➤ GET SET

Sit upright on the end of the chair or bench with your knees bent at 90 degrees and feet hip-width apart, placed securely on the floor. Also, grasp the end of the chair with palms down and knuckles facing outward. Your hands should be near your thighs, closer than shoulder-width apart.

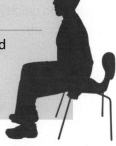

➤ GO

1. This test begins when you transfer your body weight off the chair by walking your feet out slowly and supporting your weight with your arms extended, maintaining a slight bend in your elbows.

2. Slowly and under control, bend your elbows and allow your body to move down towards the floor— go as far as you comfortably can—elbows to be no more than a 90-degree angle.

3. Next, straighten your arms, pressing from the heel of both hands, raise your body back to step 2 and repeat as many times as you can in 90 seconds. Note: If you reach 20 repetitions, you can stop the test.

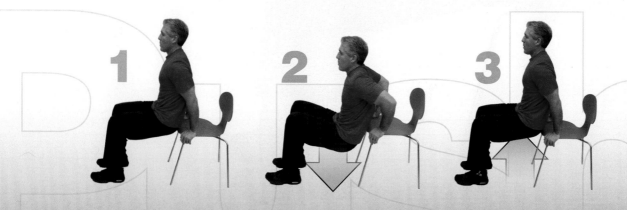

VARIATIONS

We strongly recommend warming your muscles up before performing this or any strength-training test or move. Also, if you have shoulder, elbow, lower back or wrist problems, we recommend not participating in this assessment and/or performing a variation of this assessment such as:

The Push-Up Test

Perform as many push-ups as you can (either on your knees or on your toes), touching your chin to the ground and raising back up to full extension with elbows slightly bent, and repeating as many times as you can. If you can get over 30 repetitions, you are doing very well!

YOUR SCORE

See how you did by comparing your score with the scores below. Circle how you scored.

RATING	SCORE (DIPS/REPS)
Excellent	20+
Good	15-19
Average	0-14
Fair	8-10
Poor	1-9

FAQs

How can I get the most out of my Push-Pull Moves? For best results, depending upon the form of push-pull you choose, the latest research points to performing the strengthening movements in a specific manner. Let's take a look at some of the key questions to consider when performing your push-pull at work.

How often should I perform Simple Push-Pull Moves? If you are performing light, low-repetition push-pull movements without any resistance such as body weight exercises (e.g. chair dips or push-ups), you can perform the moves daily. But, if you are performing push-pull strengthening exercises with added weights or resistance it is recommended to perform them every other day, or two to three days per week. It is recommended that you give your body 24-48 hours to properly recover after a challenging push-pull workout. You can perform the Simple Push-Pull Moves shared on pages 90–93 at work (in the office or break room, or at home). Note: Depending upon your fitness personality profile, see what might work best for you on page 98.

How hard and how many sets/reps should I perform? Factors such as your strength, muscular endurance, goals, personality and time constraints will determine the number of repetitions (or times you perform a movement) and sets (a group of repetitions) that you should complete. To help you get started with improving either your muscular strength and/or endurance using "Isotonic" training, check out these guidelines, adapted from *The American College of Sports Medicine*:

LEVEL	GOAL	INTENSITY	SETS AND REPS
Beginner	Strength	Very Light To Light Load (e.g. 40-50% of one rep maximum)	One set of 8-12 repetitions
Beginner	Endurance	Light To Moderate Load (e.g. 50% of one rep maximum)	One set of 15-20 repetitions
Intermediate	Strength	Moderate To Heavy Load (e.g. 60-70% of one rep maximum)	Two to three sets of 8-12 repetitions
Intermediate	Endurance	Light To Moderate Load (e.g. 50% of one rep maximum)	Two or more sets of 15-20 repetitions
Advanced	Strength	Hard To Very Hard Load (e.g. Above 80% of one rep maximum)	Two to four sets of 8-12 repetitions
Advanced	Endurance	Light To Moderate Load (e.g. 50% of one rep maximum)	Two or more sets of 15-20 repetitions

NOTE: The best way to improve your fitness, strength and or muscular endurance is to challenge your muscles by progressing your intensity—by increasing the number of reps, sets or resistance—as you get stronger. Remember, regardless of the type of push-pull exercises you choose to do, you should always warm up properly. Be sure to not overdo it—select a level that is appropriate for you. You can progress yourself from beginner to more challenging levels as you improve. See instructions for the Simple Push-Pull Moves on pages 90–93. Also, be sure and assess your push-pull as you practice these moves so you can see how much you improve.

NOTE: It is recommended to perform the push-pull tests on pages 94–97 every four to six weeks to see how you are improving.

It's time to test your…
Push & Pull

Now, it's time to take a look at how strong your pull muscles are.

Push-Pull Test #2: Pull-Up Test

This test is a standard in the military and one of the best assessments to determine the muscular endurance and strength of your upper back, arms, shoulders and overall fitness.

➤ GET READY

Ideally, you'll need a pull up bar (if you don't have access to one—no problem—see the *Modified Pull-Up Instructions on the next page), a pencil or pen and this book to score your results.

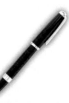

➤ GET SET

Grasp the bar with both hands, shoulder-width apart using an overhand grip (knuckles facing you), and hang from the bar so your arms are straight and your feet are off the floor, with legs bent behind you.

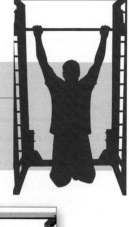

➤ GO

1. Start this test by pulling with both arms and upper back, raising your upper body up with the goal of raising your chin over the bar.

2. Lower your body down, hanging from the bar with straight arms (step 1) and repeat these steps as many times as you can without swinging, kicking, rocking or swaying.

Modification For Females: Flex-Arm Hang: Stand on a chair or bench placed underneath a pull up bar. Grasp the bar with an overhand grip and place your chin directly above the bar. Next, bend your knees and raise your feet off the chair or bench and hold as long as you can without your chin touching.

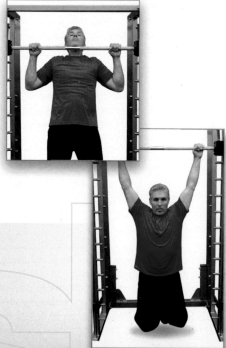

➤ FINISH

The test is completed when you:
- ✓ Are no longer able to raise your chin above the bar
- ✓ Rest your chin on the bar
- ✓ Swing, rock or kick legs to gain momentum
- ✓ Touch ground or chair with feet

VARIATIONS

Modified Pull-Up: Locate a low horizontal bar such as a handrail, or take two sturdy chairs (or a bench press/squat rack) and place a strong bar or pole between the two at hip level. Next, slide your body directly under the bar, grasping with both hands with an overhand grip. Next, straighten your legs, with your feet together and in front of you, placing the majority of your lower body weight on your heels. Position your head and chin directly under the bar. Next, perform as many modified pull-ups as you can, following steps 1-2.

Note: We strongly recommend warming your muscles up before performing this or any strength-training test or move.

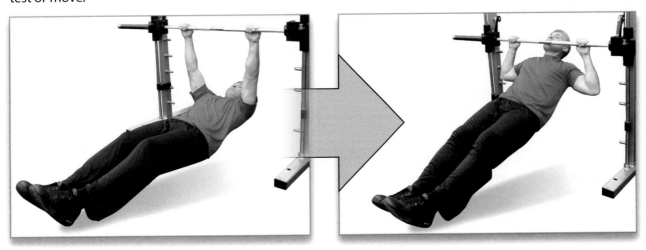

YOUR SCORE

See how you did by comparing your score with the scores below. Circle how you scored.

RATING	SCORE		
	Males (Pull-Ups)	Females (Flex-Arm Hang)	Male & Female (Modified Pull-Ups)
Excellent	13+	18+ seconds	30 and above
Good	9-13	15-18 seconds	25-29
Average	5-9	8-15 seconds	16-24
Poor	<5	<8 seconds	0-15

Push & Pull

Push-Pull Programs, Tools And Personality Profile Recommendations

To improve your push-pull, you can perform the simple movements mentioned earlier, found on pages 90–93. Or you can select from various recommended programs and tools below, based upon your Fitness That Works Personality Profile to help you with your push-pull. In the following chart, you'll see a list of recommended push-pull activities. (See specific recommendations for your Fitness Personality Profile checked in the right hand columns).

Fitness Personality Profile—My Personality Profile Is

▼   Check three that are the most appealing to you.

PUSH-PULL ACTIVITIES/EXERCISES	PROFILE A	PROFILE B	PROFILE C
☐ Simple Moves - Chair Dip (See page 90–91)	✓	✓	✓
☐ Simple Moves - Chair Shoulder Retraction Row (See page 92–93)	✓	✓	✓
☐ Reformer Machines (e.g. Pilates Studio, Allegro, Center Line, Fletcher or Sport)	✓		
☐ Elliptical Machines	✓		
☐ Cross Country Skiing Machines	✓		
☐ Dumbbells	✓		
☐ Barbells	✓		
☐ Resistance Tubing	✓		
☐ Kettle Bells	✓		
☐ Strength Resistance Machines (e.g. Bow-flex, Total Gym, Cybex, Hoist, Life Fitness)	✓		
☐ Pull-Up and Dip-Bar Towers	✓		
☐ Rowing Machines	✓		
☐ Suspension Training (e.g. TRX, FKPro or Aerosling)	✓	✓	
☐ Power or Olympic Weight Lifting	✓		
☐ Sand Bags	✓		✓
☐ Sleds	✓		
☐ Strength Fitness Classes (e.g. Circuit Classes, Boot Camps, etc...)		✓	✓
☐ Calisthenics	✓		
☐ Strength Training DVDs (e.g. 4321 Fitness, Insanity, P-90X, Body Blast)	✓		
☐ Martial Arts (e.g. Judo, Jujutsu, Kung Fu, Mixed Martial Arts, Jeet Kune Do, Taekwondo)	✓	✓	
☐ Gymnastics Classes (Bars/Rings)		✓	
☐ Rock Climbing			✓
☐ Rowing (Scull Club Racing)		✓	✓
☐ Cross Country Skiing			✓
☐ Surfing (Paddling)		✓	✓
☐ Canoeing		✓	✓
☐ Kayaking		✓	✓
☐ Wrestling (Greco & Freestyle)		✓	✓
☐ 4-3-2-1 Fitness Training (See pages 148–149)	✓	✓	✓

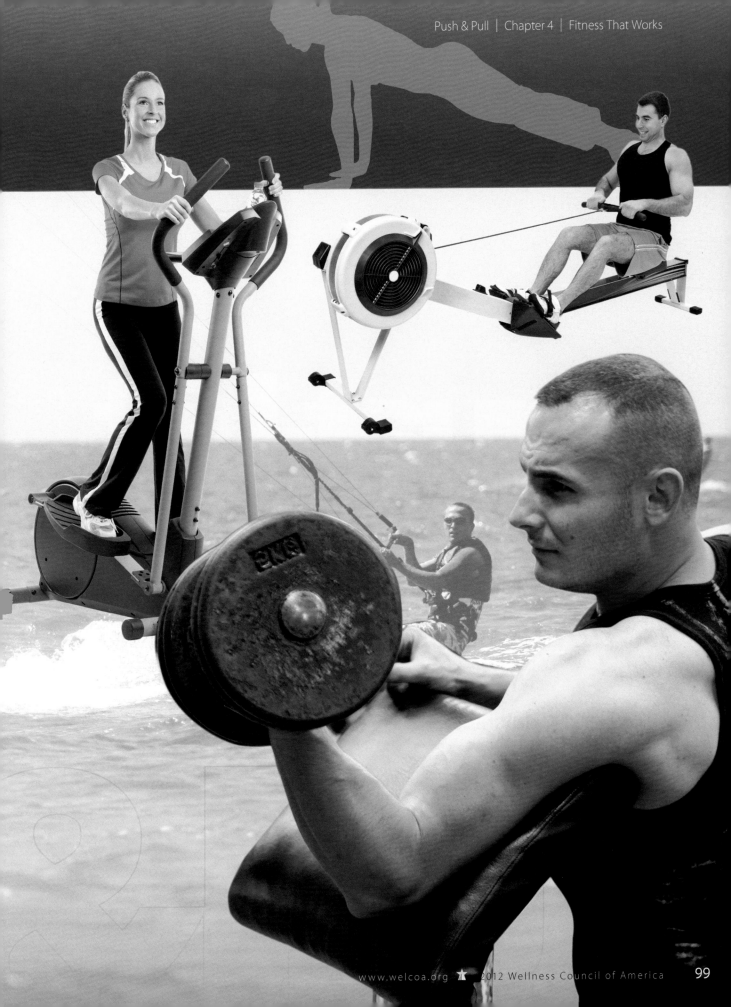

Squat-Lift

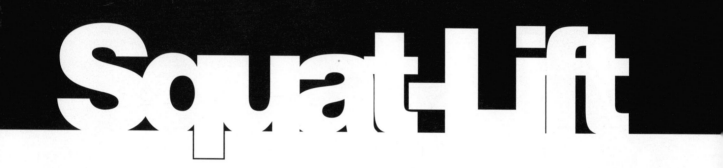

"Whenever I feel like exercise, I lie down until the feeling passes."

—Robert M. Hutchins

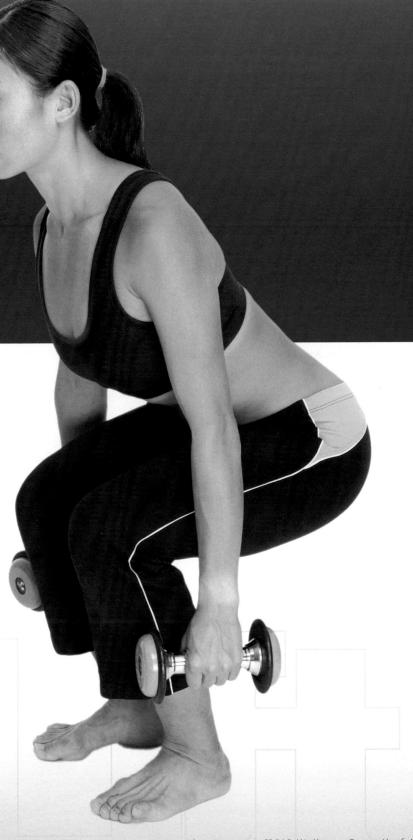

Squat-Lift

CONGRATULATIONS! TODAY IS YOUR "DAY OF REST." TAKE A MINUTE TO PICTURE YOURSELF RECLINING ON YOUR SOFA OR EASY CHAIR WITH YOUR FAVORITE BOOK OR THE TV REMOTE, READY TO ENJOY YOUR DAY OF DOING ABSOLUTELY NOTHING. A DAY AWAY FROM ALL THE HUSTLE AND BUSTLE—JUST SOME TIME FOR SERIOUS "R AND R." AH, ISN'T THIS THE LIFE?

What if you could take your day of rest and turn it into two days or three days or a week, or better yet a month? What if you could parlay this experience into a year of doing absolutely nothing physically; not having to move a muscle? Have you ever thought about what it would be like if you threw the idea of physical activity and exercise away for a while?

Wow, what would it be like? For one month or one year, picture no sweating. No sore muscles. No waking up early or time taken away from the family or work. No worrying about what to wear at the gym. No feeling guilty about missing that walk you promised yourself to do. No… (you fill in the blank).

Ask yourself: "What would it be like if I didn't exercise for a week, a month or a year? What would change?"

How would life be different? How would you be different?

In this chapter, I'd like to take you on a tour of two different lifestyles: one that's filled with leisure and inactivity, and the other filled with movement and activity throughout your day. My goal is to allow you the opportunity to weigh the pros and cons, and make your own decision about the type of life which appeals to you. In this chapter, I'll be laying out the benefits of our fifth simple move, "squat-lift," and how performing it on a regular basis may be just the thing to help you get off—and stay off—the couch.

We will explore:

1 What is squat-lift?

2 Why squat-lift is so important

3 How inactivity impacts your squat-lift

4 Simple moves you can do to improve your squat-lift

5 How to test your squat-lift

6 Recommended squat-lift programs, tools and much more

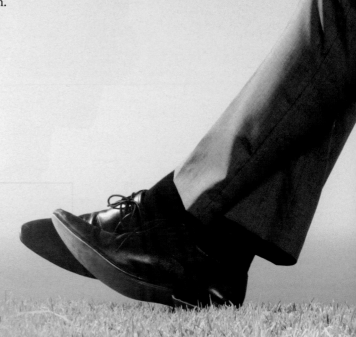

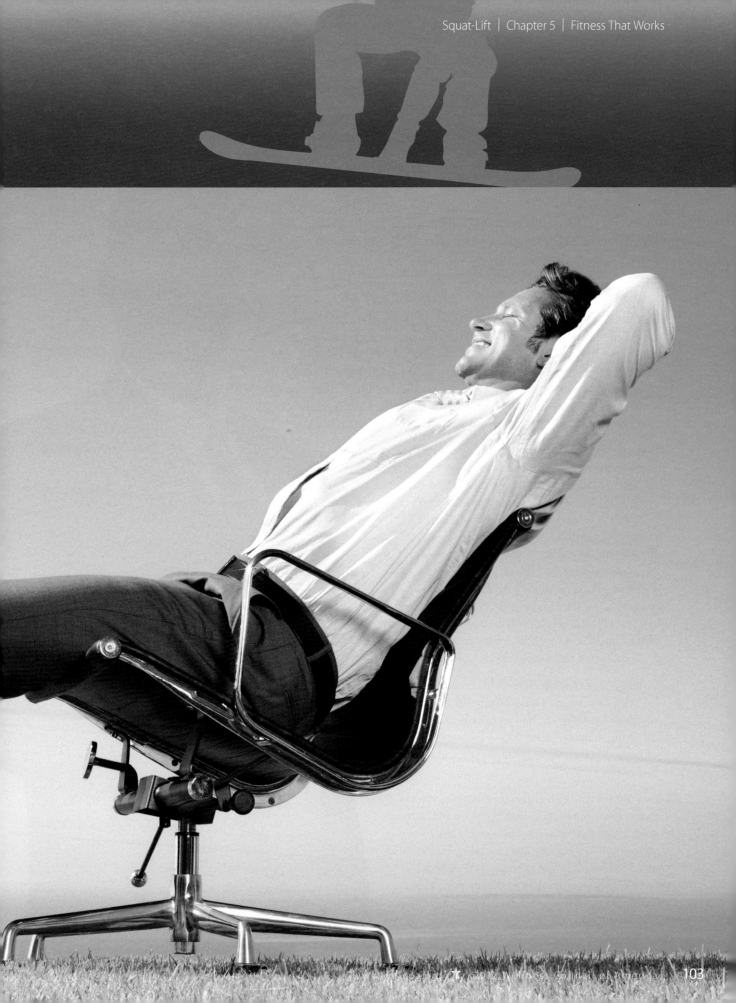

Squat-Lift

How To Cure "Gluteal Amnesia:"

"Boy, do you look old!" Greg shouted to his co-worker and old college buddy, Mark. Just like the good old days, Mark and Greg shook hands and quickly embraced. "How are you Mark?" asked Greg. "It's been way too long, my friend." The two smiled and continued to shake hands.

Greg and Mark had been inseparable since they were in elementary school. They went to the same high school and then college, where they played football together over 20 years ago. Now, they both worked for the same large manufacturing company in Orange County, California. Oddly, it had been a number of months since they had seen one another because Mark had been promoted to a new position and was traveling quite a bit. Now, seeing each other for the first time in a while, they had plenty of catching up to do.

Both were approaching their late 40s and each of the men had been noticing some significant differences in their mid-life experience. Mark said, "You know, Greg, you tease, but I do feel old! I don't know what's going on. I need to find a way to get back in shape. My belly's started hanging over my belt, my legs and back ache all the time, and do you know what my teenage son said to me the other day? He said, 'Dad, you don't have a butt anymore!'" Mark then turned around to show Greg his backside. "I look like a 90 year old from behind," Mark laughed, then added, "But look at you. You look the same as you did in college. What in the world are you doing?"

Smiling, Greg chuckled and hit his friend on the shoulder. "You've got 'Gluteal Amnesia,' bud! Your butt has forgotten how to work because you are sitting so much," Greg teased, but only half jokingly. "Partner, we've got to get you and your butt back!"

Greg shared that he had also been noticing the same things about five months ago: "I just felt old, achy, tired, weak, soft, fat—you name it, my body was going south in a big way and in a hurry. Funny thing was, I found out I wasn't the only one. A bunch of other middle-aged guys in our department were feeling the same way too. So we decided as a group to begin moving more throughout the day. The company offered us training on how to sit less during the day and showed us some 'Simple Moves' we can do during the day and at home. We have been blown away at how much better we all look and feel since we started!" Greg happily reported.

Mark was all ears as Greg shared what his team had been doing together over the last few months. Mark asked how he could participate and discovered that he could share the "Simple Moves" workouts with his department—and even perform them while traveling by himself, or at home. After a few months of leading his own group at work and moving more even while traveling, Mark has been thrilled to see a personal change as well changes among his team members. The good news is that Mark and Greg are now both back to the same fit, healthy, playing-weights that they were in college. And best of all (at least according to Mark's son), is that through this process, Mark got his butt back!

"If you could bottle everything you get from physical activity and sell it at a pharmacy, it would go for a hefty price."
—George Sheehan, MD

What Is Squat-Lift?

Think about all the activities you perform throughout your workday that involve squatting and lifting. From bending down to lift up a light object off the ground such as a pencil, set of keys or small change, or larger items such as a briefcase, bucket, heavy package or even weighted machinery, all of these movements require the ability, strength, flexibility and coordination to squat down and lift an object safely.

Squat: The simple motion of squatting is to bend your knees and sit down into a crouching position. Lift: The motion of "lift," according to multiple dictionary and biomechanical references, is simply to raise or move something from a lower position to a higher position. Squat + Lift = "Squat-Lift." Put them together and you have one fluid motion with two actions requiring multiple muscle groups from lower and upper body to work in coordination with one another, lowering your body down and then up—helping you move an object to its desired location.

3 SIMPLE REASONS TO SQUAT-LIFT

Considered by many researchers and trainers to be one of the best exercises to perform during your workday, here are three simple reasons to squat-lift:

1. **Get the best bang for your exercise buck!** The squat-lift is rated one of the best exercises for total body fitness because it works so many muscles at one time (for example, your legs, hips, buttocks, core, lower and upper back, shoulders neck and arms) in just one motion. Try and achieve that with a bicep curl!

2. **Increase metabolism and burn body fat.** According to researchers such as Wayne Westcott PhD, performing total body resistance training movements such as the squat-lift will help increase metabolism, reduce unwanted body fat and increase lean muscle.

3. **Prevent gluteal amnesia by shaping and toning your butt, back and legs.** According to inactivity researchers, the more we sit, the faster we lose one of the largest and strongest muscles of our body: our buttocks or gluteus maximus. When weakened, the lack of this muscle puts more pressure on other muscles (such as our hips and lower back) and limits our ability to work efficiently. Also, a glute that is disappearing lowers metabolism and impacts weight gain. According to researchers, the squat-lift is one of the best movements to help prevent this 'gluteal amnesia,' improving metabolism, tone and strengthening the entire lower body.

Squat-Lift

The Goal Of Squat-Lift

The goal with the motion of squat-lift is simple: to help strengthen your lower and upper body, while training you to correctly and efficiently lift objects in a way that minimizes injury throughout your work day and life.

How To Improve Your Squat-Lift

Since the squat-lift is a resistance training motion, as we discussed in the push-pull section (Chapter 4), you can review the benefits of these two types of training (Isotonic and Isometric) again on pages 86-87.

How Inactivity Impacts Your Squat-Lift

Take a seat. Picture yourself sitting down for the big game (or favorite TV show) in an over sized, luxurious, dark brown leather chair. As you begin to snuggle into the rich, deep, back pillows, you notice something a little different with this particular chair. If you lift your left arm, underneath it you'll find…drum roll please…you guessed it, a mini refrigerator stocked with your favorite treats, snacks and drinks. While this may sound like fiction, this particular piece of furniture is known as the "Cool Chair," and is a best-seller for one of the largest chair and sofa manufacturers in the world. Wow! We now can sit back with our remote control in one hand to change channels, and enjoy ice cream, soda or beer from right underneath us as we watch the Super Bowl! We won't have to move an inch! (Except to go to the bathroom, maybe… If only they could invent a "Port-a-Potty" chair—an invention, which I'm sure, is not too far off!)

While inventions over the years, such as the TV, elevators, escalators and now the "Cool Chair" have been blamed for soaring obesity statistics over the last few decades, recent research now points to an additional culprit which may be even more dangerous to our ever expanding waist-lines and declining health and fitness. What is it?

Sitting Down On The Job!

Researchers point out the modern sedentary American workplace (or what has been referred to as a "desk sentence"), may contribute more to the decline of our health and fitness than we ever imagined. Researchers are beginning to understand the impact this type of "sedentary work-style" has on one's health and life. (See the side bar about sitting versus squatting-lifting on page 107).

According to Barbara E. Ainsworth, an exercise researcher from the American College of Sports Medicine, "I think occupational activity is part of that missing puzzle that is so difficult to measure, and is probably contributing to the inactivity and creeping obesity that we're seeing over time." Dr. James Levine, also an expert in the field of inactivity and health from the Mayo Clinic, has determined that how individuals spend their work day can have a dramatic impact upon their waist-line, metabolism, calorie burning, health and longevity. According to Dr. Levine, the average American employee spends the majority of their time seated. Estimates range from seven to eight hours per day at their desk or at lunch as well as an additional five to six hours seated while commuting, watching TV or on their computer seated at home. Dr. Levine states from his research, "Excessive sitting is a lethal activity."

But there is hope. According to Levine, small movements performed throughout one's day (such as the Simple Moves we have been discussing in this book: squat-lift, reach, step and others) can significantly thwart the decline to one's health and creeping weight gains. What Dr. Levine refers to as NEAT: Non-Exercise Activity Thermogenesis, or non-sweat activities can be performed throughout your day to help you expend much more energy. Such NEAT activities can have an even greater impact on your health than visiting the gym after work! The best part is that doing these simple movements throughout your day only requires subtle changes to your daily work routine. NEAT exercises have been found to:

- ✓ Burn more calories than a half-hour running on a treadmill;
- ✓ Reduce fatigue by 65%;
- ✓ Lower blood pressure;
- ✓ Enhance creativity;
- ✓ Lower body weight;
- ✓ Improve muscle memory, tone and metabolism;
- ✓ Decrease stress;
- ✓ Increase productivity;
- ✓ And much, much more.

WHAT HAPPENS TO OUR BODIES WHEN WE SIT TOO MUCH?

Should I or shouldn't I? That is the question. Sit or squat? Leisure or lift? Should I really be concerned about "sitting" too much? Or should I take a little time to do a few squat-lifts? Is it really worth it to move my body with Simple Moves periodically throughout the day? The answer is, YES! According to the latest scientific research, the physiological and psychological effects of sitting too long and too much throughout your day significantly diminish the quality of your health and fitness. Just a minute or two of Simple Moves can drastically impact your personal well-being. The following chart illustrates the stark contrast of the effects of sitting too much versus the effects when you're moving throughout your day.

Note: All items with a (+) indicate an increase and all items with a (–) indicate a decrease in each of the particular health or fitness benefits.

	Sitting (From 9 to 5 pm)	Squatting/Lifting (Simple Moves performed periodically from 9 to 5 pm)
Metabolism and fat burning enzymes	–	+
Body fat	+	–
Muscle-strength, size and tone	–	+
Ligaments, tendons and bone strength	–	+
Back and core strength	–	+
Cardiovascular health	–	+
Energy	–	+
Cholesterol and triglycerides	+	–
Coordination and balance	–	+
Creativity	–	+
Productivity	–	+
Stress, depression and anxiety	+	–
Self-esteem and self-image	–	+

Squat-Lift

YOUR SITTING JOURNAL

How physically active are you in your job? One of the most effective ways to diagnose if you have "Sitting Disease" is to track the amount of time you spend sitting down. Take a moment to determine how much time you spend on your rump, seated. As discussed, recent research is pointing to the impact that sitting throughout the day can have on your personal health and fitness.

Use this form to track the amount of time you spend sitting at work. Be sure to include your commute time as well as lunch and/or break time that you are seated during your day.

Monitor your sitting at work for one week and then do the math: Average total # of hours per day spent sitting down _____ × 5 = _____ (This is your average total # of hours per week / work week spent sitting down). Now take your average total # of hours per week (work week) spent sitting down × 4 = _____ (This is your average total # of hours per month spent sitting down).

Daily Sitting Scores

Rating	Time Spent Sitting
Excellent	Below 1-2 hours a day along with very active/physical labor during day
Good	2-3 hours a day with moderate movements during day
Average	4-5 hours per day with some light movements during day
Poor	6 or more hours per day with no movement during day

If you scored in the average or poor category, consider the list below to help you move throughout your day.

"Do This —Not That" During Your Work Day

"Do This"	"Not That"
Stand or pace when talking on the phone	Sit when talking on the phone
Take the stairs	Take the elevator
Set your phone alarm to signal you to perform a Simple Move every 30 or 60 minutes (e.g. 10 squat-lifts, or balance moves or reach moves).	Sit all day without moving or taking breaks
Fidget when on the phone	Sit still when on the phone
Take a "walk and talk" meeting with colleagues	Sit down when holding meetings
Stand when doing desk work—place computer on higher table or book case	Sit when performing computer or office work
Take a standing break every 30-60 minutes (stand for 5-10 minutes)	Sit down when drinking coffee or taking a break
Walk fast to copy or coffee machine	Send someone else do to your copying or get your coffee
Stand up and walk to speak or deliver a message to colleagues	Email or text colleagues

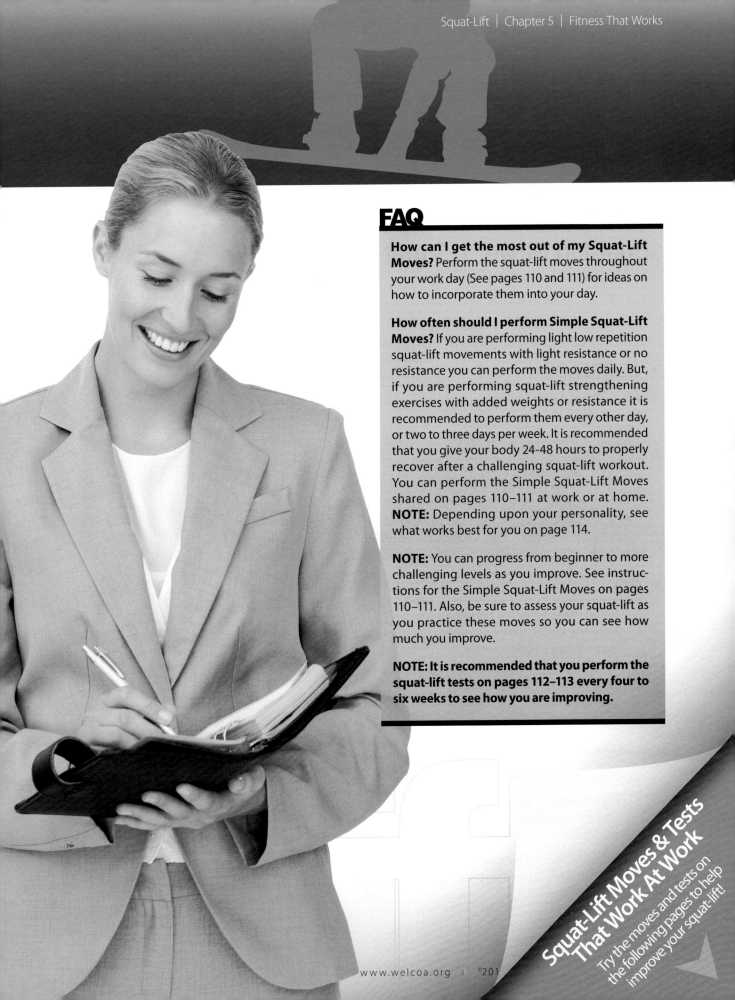

FAQ

How can I get the most out of my Squat-Lift Moves? Perform the squat-lift moves throughout your work day (See pages 110 and 111) for ideas on how to incorporate them into your day.

How often should I perform Simple Squat-Lift Moves? If you are performing light low repetition squat-lift movements with light resistance or no resistance you can perform the moves daily. But, if you are performing squat-lift strengthening exercises with added weights or resistance it is recommended to perform them every other day, or two to three days per week. It is recommended that you give your body 24-48 hours to properly recover after a challenging squat-lift workout. You can perform the Simple Squat-Lift Moves shared on pages 110–111 at work or at home. **NOTE:** Depending upon your personality, see what works best for you on page 114.

NOTE: You can progress from beginner to more challenging levels as you improve. See instructions for the Simple Squat-Lift Moves on pages 110–111. Also, be sure to assess your squat-lift as you practice these moves so you can see how much you improve.

NOTE: It is recommended that you perform the squat-lift tests on pages 112–113 every four to six weeks to see how you are improving.

Squat-Lift Moves & Tests That Work At Work

Try the moves and tests on the following pages to help improve your squat-lift!

It's time to improve your...
Squat-Lift

It's time to move...

Squat-Lift Move #1: Squat-Lift (With Water Bottle)

This simple move is a very effective way to strengthen your upper and lower body, core, and improve your mobility. It also helps train your body to lift objects correctly. The best part of this move is that you can perform it during work—in your office, manufacturing area and break-room, or even at home—with or without an object to lift.

➤ GET READY

All you'll need is a non-slip surface to stand on and a full, 16 ounce plastic water bottle.

➤ GET SET

Stand with your feet slightly wider than shoulder width apart and toes pointed out slightly. With both arms extended and hands positioned below your waist, hold the top of a full 16 ounce plastic water bottle with both hands, placed in between your thighs.

➤ GO

1. Begin the exercise by bending from the knees, lowering down into a squat position, while keeping your hands and arms (and water bottle) in between your thighs.

2. Touch the ground with the bottom of the water bottle while keeping your torso upright and chest up.

3. Repeat steps 1 and 2, eight to 20 times or as many as you can safely complete.

NOTE: If you have severe back or knee problems, it is recommended that you modify this move.

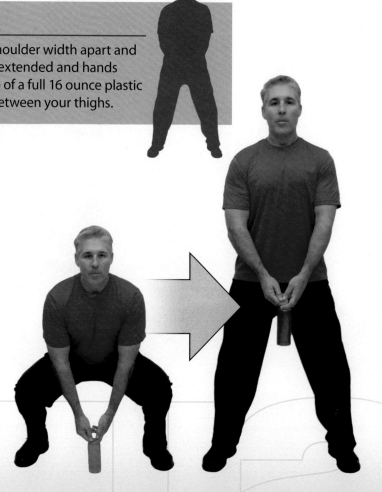

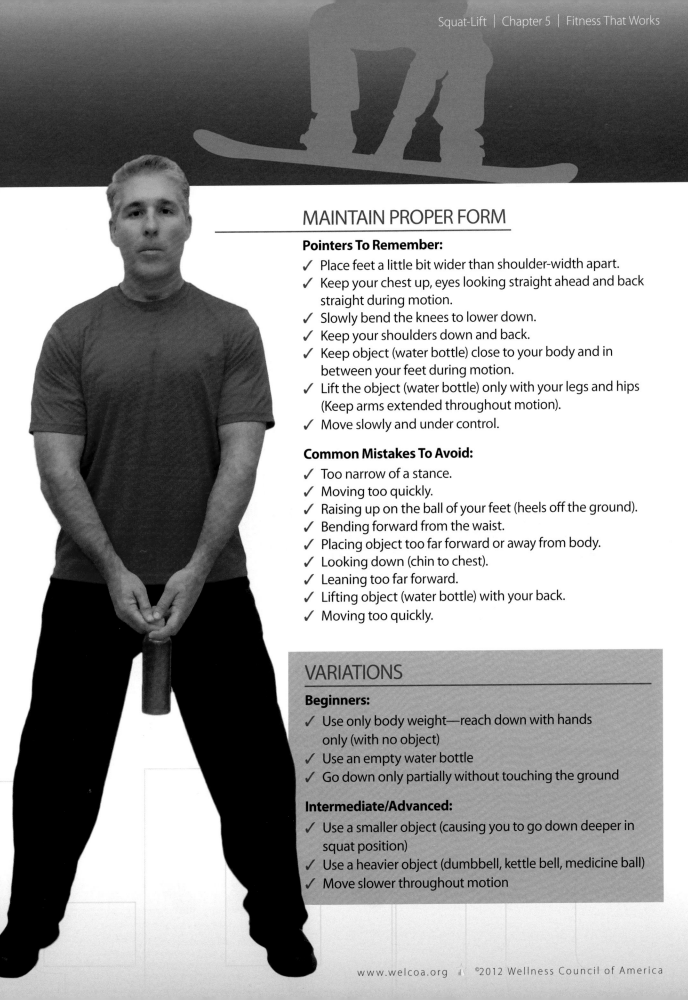

MAINTAIN PROPER FORM

Pointers To Remember:

✓ Place feet a little bit wider than shoulder-width apart.
✓ Keep your chest up, eyes looking straight ahead and back straight during motion.
✓ Slowly bend the knees to lower down.
✓ Keep your shoulders down and back.
✓ Keep object (water bottle) close to your body and in between your feet during motion.
✓ Lift the object (water bottle) only with your legs and hips (Keep arms extended throughout motion).
✓ Move slowly and under control.

Common Mistakes To Avoid:

✓ Too narrow of a stance.
✓ Moving too quickly.
✓ Raising up on the ball of your feet (heels off the ground).
✓ Bending forward from the waist.
✓ Placing object too far forward or away from body.
✓ Looking down (chin to chest).
✓ Leaning too far forward.
✓ Lifting object (water bottle) with your back.
✓ Moving too quickly.

VARIATIONS

Beginners:

✓ Use only body weight—reach down with hands only (with no object)
✓ Use an empty water bottle
✓ Go down only partially without touching the ground

Intermediate/Advanced:

✓ Use a smaller object (causing you to go down deeper in squat position)
✓ Use a heavier object (dumbbell, kettle bell, medicine ball)
✓ Move slower throughout motion

It's time to test your...

Squat-Lift

Now that you've practiced your Squat-Lift Moves that Work At Work, let's take a moment to see how mobile and strong your lower body muscles are.

Test #1: Squat-Lift Test

Having a strong and functional lower body is essential to completing daily tasks throughout your workday, as well as keeping you healthy and fit. To test the muscular endurance and strength of your lower body, let me introduce you to the Squat-Lift Test. This test measures your mobility and the muscular endurance of your thighs, hamstrings, gluteus maximus, back, shoulders and arms.

➤ GET READY

You'll need a non-slip surface to stand on, a full, 16 ounce plastic water bottle, a timing device such as a stopwatch, wristwatch or cell phone, a pencil or pen and this book to score your results.

➤ GET SET

Stand with feet slightly wider than shoulder-width apart and toes pointed out slightly. With both arms extended and hands positioned below your waist, hold the top of a full, 16 ounce plastic water bottle with both hands, placed in between your thighs.

➤ GO

1. Begin the test by bending from the knees, lowering down into a squat position, while keeping your hands and arms (and water bottle) in between your thighs.

2. Touch the ground with the bottom of the water bottle while keeping your torso upright and chest up.

3. Repeat steps 1 and 2 as many times as you can in one minute and write down your total number of repetitions.

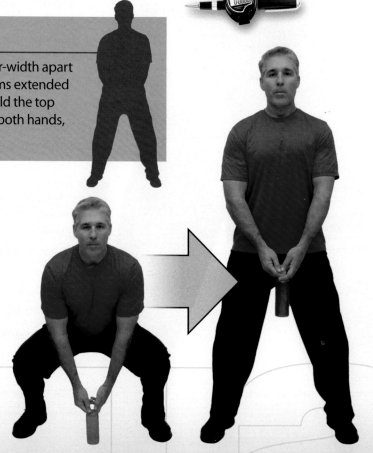

FINISH

The test is completed when:

✓ One minute has expired.

✓ You bend too far forward from the waist to touch the water bottle to the ground.

✓ You cannot touch the ground with the water bottle.

✓ One hand comes off of the water bottle.

✓ You experience discomfort or pain in lower back or knees.

OPTIONAL

If you cannot touch the ground with the water bottle, place a chair behind you and perform as many squats as you can in one minute, touching your buttocks lightly to the chair with each squat.

We strongly recommend warming up your muscles before performing this or any strength-training test or move. Also, if you have lower back, knee or hip problems, we recommend not participating in this assessment.

YOUR SCORE

See how you did by comparing your score with the scores below. Circle how you scored.

RATING	SCORE
Excellent	25+ repetitions
Good	20-24 repetitions
Average	11-19 repetitions
Poor	1-10 repetitions

Squat-Lift

Squat-Lift Programs, Tools And Personality Profile Recommendations

To improve your squat-lift, you can perform simple movements like those mentioned on pages 110–111. Or, select squat-lift activities from this chart containing various recommended programs and tools based upon your Fitness That Works Personality Profile. Note: All programs, tools or activities that are checked are recommended for you.

Fitness Personality Profile—My Personality Profile Is

▼ Check three that are the most appealing to you.

PUSH-PULL ACTIVITIES/EXERCISES	PROFILE A	PROFILE B	PROFILE C
☐ Simple Moves - Squat-Lift (See page 110–111)	✓	✓	✓
☐ Dumbbells, barbells, or free weights	✓		
☐ Medicine Ball	✓		
☐ Resistance Tubing	✓		
☐ Kettle Bell	✓		
☐ Tire Flipping	✓		
☐ Sledgehammer	✓		
☐ Wood Chopping	✓		✓
☐ Strength Resistance Machines (e.g. Bow-flex, Total Gym, Cybex, Hoist, Life Fitness)	✓		
☐ Suspension Training (e.g. TRX, FKPro or Aerosling)	✓	✓	
☐ Power or Olympic Weight Lifting	✓		
☐ Sand Bags	✓		✓
☐ Strength Fitness Classes (e.g. Circuit Classes, Boot Camps, etc.)		✓	✓
☐ Strong Man/Woman Competitions (Squat/Dead Lifts)	✓		
☐ Strength Training DVDs (e.g. 4321 Fitness, Insanity, P-90X, Body Blast)	✓		
☐ Martial Arts (e.g. Judo, Mixed Martial Arts, Jeet Kune Do, Taekwondo)	✓	✓	
☐ Fencing		✓	✓
☐ Softball/Baseball		✓	✓
☐ Dance (Ballet)		✓	
☐ Water Skiing		✓	✓
☐ Snowboarding or Snow Skiing		✓	✓
☐ Basketball		✓	✓
☐ Wrestling (Sumo, Free Style, Greco)		✓	✓
☐ Football (Flag or Tackle)		✓	✓
☐ Rugby		✓	✓
☐ 4–3–2–1 Fitness Training (See page 148–149)	✓	✓	✓

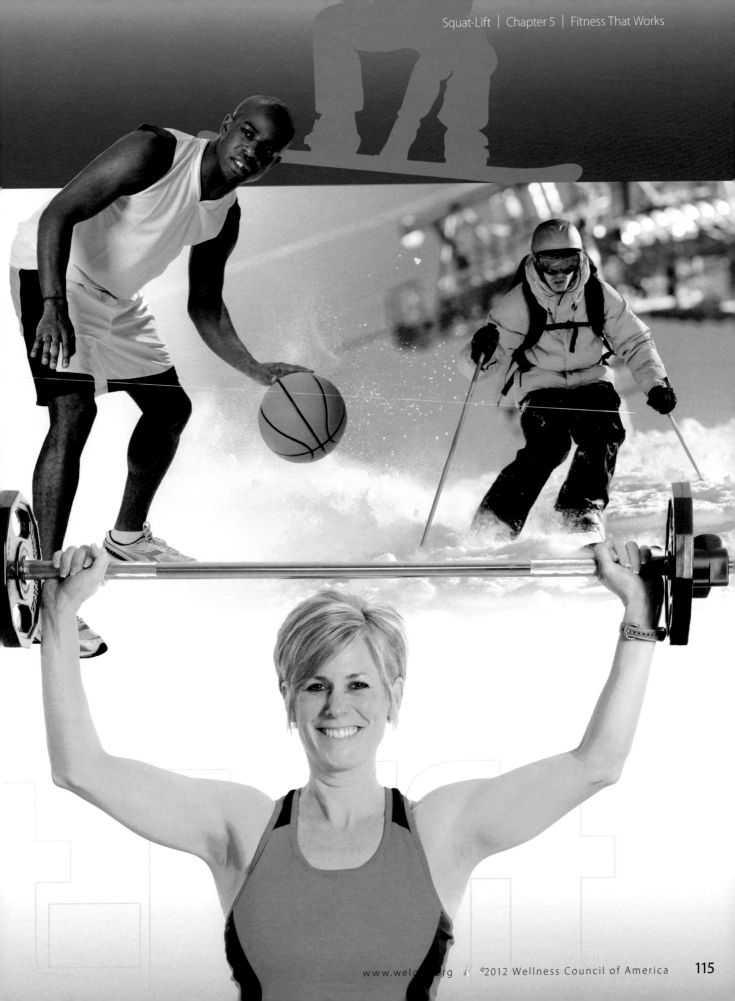

Twist

"Come on baby, let's do the twist
Come on baby, let's do the twist
Take me by my hand and go like this..."

—"The Twist" Lyrics by Chubby Checker

Twist

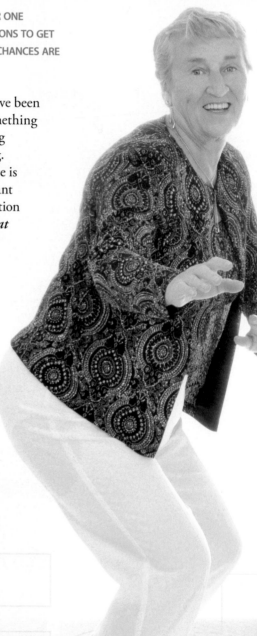

In THE 1960'S, AMERICAN SINGER AND SONG WRITER CHUBBY CHECKER'S NUMBER ONE SELLING SONG CREATED A DANCE CRAZE ACROSS THE NATION PROMPTING MILLIONS TO GET UP OUT OF THEIR SEATS AND "DO THE TWIST!" IF YOU HAVE EVER HEARD THE SONG, CHANCES ARE IT PUT A SMILE ON YOUR FACE, A TAP IN YOUR TOES AND GOT YOU DANCING TOO.

Hmmm? What if we thought of exercise in the same light? Most of us have been taught by health professionals to think of exercising as a discipline or something that we should do, but rarely do we think of exercise as a joy or something that we want to do. But here's a twist, the song and message are changing. According to the U.S. Surgeon General, Regina Benjamin, MD, "Exercise is the new medicine. It will make you feel a lot better." She continues, "I want to move from a negative conversation about disease to a positive conversation about being healthy and fit. *We need to stop bombarding people with what they can't do and start talking about what they enjoy doing.*" What a refreshing way to look at exercise—what we want to do instead of what we have to do.

In this chapter, we are going to look at fitness with a little twist. I'll be showing you how much fun you can have with our sixth move, "twist," and how performing it on a regular basis just may bring a smile to your face and a tap to your toes!

We will explore:

1   What is twist?

2   Why twist is so important

3   How to look and feel years younger

4   Simple moves you can do to improve your twist

5   How to test your twist

6   Recommended twist programs, tools and much more

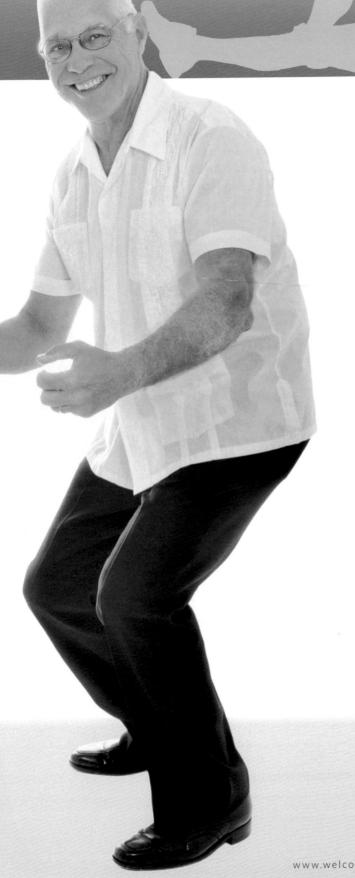

"We need to stop bombarding people with what they can't do and start talking about what they enjoy doing."

Twist

Get Your Joy Back!

"I've spent the last few years trying to get back in shape, but I just can't seem to muster the motivation to make it happen!" said Marie. We had been meeting over the last few weeks talking about her goals and desires for her health and fitness, and she began to share how the last few years had been difficult. "I just kind of feel numb, like I am going through the motions with everything in my life. My kids are busy with high school and getting ready to go off to college, my husband's job is so busy we don't see each other as often as we'd like and I'm caretaking for my elderly father-in-law. I know I need to exercise and eat healthy, but sitting on the couch after a long day and eating chocolate ice cream feels a lot better." I could see the pain in Marie's eyes as she shared her struggles.

After a short break in the conversation, I asked her, "Marie, what brings you joy?" She looked at me with a strange expression. "Joy? What's joy got to do with working out?" I told her since she had been through quite a bit of stress over the last few years, the last thing she needed was someone (like me) to tell her to do something she didn't want to do—and that she needed to find her joy. "Well, it definitely isn't exercise, if that's what you are trying to make me say." I smiled and assured her I wasn't trying to trick her. "No, forget about exercise. What is something you really enjoy doing? Something that brings a smile to your face?" I said. She thought for a moment, "Let's see, besides chocolate, coffee, a good movie or hanging out with my family and friends….I love birds, music and dancing!" I said, "Ok, do you remember a time when you experienced this joy to the fullest?" She paused again and said, "When I was a teenager I used to sit and listen to music 'til late at night. It would take me to a different place. Sometimes I would just dance in my room all by myself. I loved that time. Then as I grew older, my husband and I used to go to concerts or go dancing when we were dating. It was so much fun! But after we had been married for a bit and the kids came along, busyness, work, stress—you know—life happened and I just seemed to put 'it' and 'me' on the shelf."

We chatted for a bit longer and I asked Marie to think of other activities or hobbies she'd be willing to try that would bring her joy this week. She looked at me again and said, "No diet or exercise, right? Just something that makes me experience joy?" I nodded and she smiled.

The next week, Marie came back and shared how much fun she had using her daughter's iPod and listening to her favorite music when driving, at

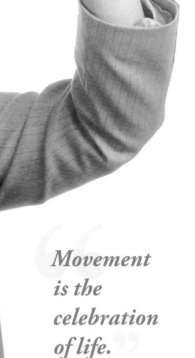

work and almost everywhere she went. Marie said she had a smile on her face and a song in her heart the entire week. She looked at me and said, "Guess what? I'm going to start dancing again too!" I smiled and asked her, "Where are you going to start dancing?" Marie then proudly reported, "I'm joining a country line dancing class at the local community center and I'm not stopping there—I'm going to start dancing at work too. A group of us from the office are already talking about learning how to belly dance!" She said with a wink. Then she moved closer to me, "I know what you are thinking…just for your information, I am not exercising. I'm just dancing and having fun!" I smiled, gave her a high five and told her, "Marie, it looks like you're on your way to get your joy back." She nodded and did a little two-step!

What Is Twist?

Dictionaries define "twist" in the following ways: "to cause to move with a turning motion" or "to turn so as to face another direction." Regardless of the definition selected, the motion twist is something we all do every day. If you think about your day yesterday, chances are you performed the motion of twist when turning to get up out of bed, getting in and out of your car, looking over your shoulder, swiveling in your chair to grab a folder file, or if you had some "fun time," you may have even swung a golf club, baseball bat, tennis or racquetball racket. All of these twist activities require multiple muscle groups and actions to work in coordination with one another. For example, you need the appropriate amount of strength from your oblique (or waist muscles), abdominal and back muscles along with the necessary flexibility and mobility of your spine to accomplish these and other twist motions.

> *Movement is the celebration of life.*
>
> —John Selland

GETTING YOUR JOY BACK

It's been estimated that the average child laughs over 300 times a day and the average adult only 10-15 times. Why is this? Stress, work demands and all the pressures of life can slowly chip away at our joy. To help get your joy back, take a moment to consider the following questions:

- When you were a child, what activities or hobbies brought you the most joy?

- What brings you joy now as an adult?

- Make a list of your top five "joy-filled" activities, games, sports or hobbies.

- How would you rate your current level of joy?
  Low   Medium   High

- What are you willing to try from your list above to bring more joy to your life?

Twist

The Goal Of Twist

The primary goal with the motion of twist is simple: To have FUN by showing you some simple moves that will bring a smile to your face. Other goals are to strengthen your waist, abdominal and back muscles (creating a "natural girdle" for your body), and improve the flexibility and mobility of your back while training you to correctly move your body in such a way that minimizes injury when twisting during your work activities or daily life.

How To Improve Your Twist

Since the twist motion is a flexibility and mobility movement like those we have previously discussed (see Reach, Chapter 2) as well as a resistance training motion (see Push-Pull, Chapter 4), you can review the benefits of these two types of training again on pages 43–45 and 86–87.

How To Look And Feel Years Younger:

Picture yourself when you were nine or ten years old. It's a warm summer day, the birds are chirping, and you don't have a care in the world other than what you are going to do for the day. Do you remember those long summer days filled with endless hours of activities, such as running, jumping, swimming, skipping, skateboarding, roller skating, or playing tag, catch, or hide and seek? They were all filled with laughter, fun and great joy. For most of us, playing was a natural part of our everyday lives. We didn't even know we were exercising because we were just having so much fun. The same is possible today. We just need to be intentional about it.

Carol Torgan, a representative of the American College of Sports Medicine, recommends the following approach: "Think of activities you liked as a kid, such as jumping rope, taking a hike, riding your bike, tossing a Frisbee, or playing hopscotch or kickball. They're good for your mind, body, and soul."

Shannon Slovensky, MEd, an exercise physiologist with the University of Virginia Health System has found: "The main idea is to find something you enjoy, because then you'll be more likely to do it! Exercise doesn't have to be a formal class at the gym and you don't need to hire a personal trainer to get in shape. Just make moving fun, and over time, you'll notice a difference in the way you look and feel."

According to Slovensky and other "play" oriented fitness experts, moving your body and playing throughout your work day not only enhances your creativity and productivity, but it can also help bring your joy back. Here are five tips to help you look and feel years younger:

1   **Dance!** Set the tone: Download your favorite "joy-filled" tune (e.g. "The Twist" by Chubby Checker) and make it your ring tone on your cell phone. Set it to go off every hour. This can serve as a reminder for you to get up and dance (or move) on the hour, or every time someone calls you. It's sure to put a smile on your face (and on those around you).

2   **Play with toys:** Create a "toy box" at work filled with jump ropes, hula-hoops, Frisbees, balloons and balls to play with throughout your day. Once you begin tossing a ball or jumping rope during break times, others will want to come out and play too.

3   **Laugh and inspire:** Throughout your day, get up from your desk or work station and share a quick joke or inspirational quote with others in your office or work environment. It'll get you up and moving, and you'll bring some joy to those around you!

4   **Challenge:** If you're the social type, consider enlisting others to join you in fitness competitions and/ or games throughout your day (e.g. How many times did you get up from your desk today and dance? How many stairs did you climb today?).

5   **Play outdoors:** If possible, go outside on breaks or at lunchtime and breathe in some fresh air while you enjoy some "simple moves" and some sunshine. This is also a good time to think about what has brought you joy during your day.

Twist Moves & Twist Tests That Work At Work
Try the moves and tests on the following pages to help improve your twist!

It's time to improve your…
Twist

Now, try this move…

Twist Move #1: Standing Twist (With Water Bottle)

This simple move is a very effective way to strengthen your waist, abs, back, shoulders and arms, as well as improve the flexibility and mobility of your back. Like all the other moves you have learned throughout this book, you can perform this twist motion during work—from 9 to 5 in your office, manufacturing area, break-room, while you travel or even at home—with or without an object to twist with.

➤ GET READY

All you'll need is a non-slip surface to stand on, and if you'd like, a full 16 ounce plastic water bottle.

➤ GET SET

Stand with your feet a little wider than shoulder-width apart with knees slightly bent, both arms extended and hands positioned at waist level, holding a full 16 ounce plastic water bottle with interlocked fingers.

➤ GO

1. Begin the exercise by tightening your abdominal muscles and slowly twisting or rotating your torso to your right, while keeping your hands and arms (and water bottle) near waist level. Stop when you feel your waist muscles tighten.

2. Twist back to the other side while keeping your abs tight and hips forward.

3. Repeat steps 1 and 2, eight to 20 times or as many as you can safely complete.

NOTE: It is important when performing this twisting motion not to over-extend or rotate too far, or too quickly, as this may cause discomfort in your lower back. Also, if you have back problems it is recommended that you not perform this exercise and I would encourage you to either modify this move or select a different abdominal/waist exercise.

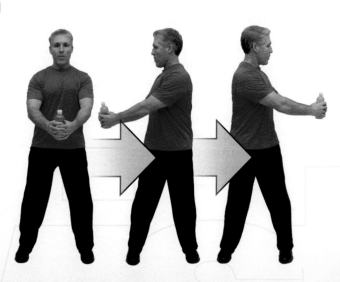

MAINTAIN PROPER FORM

Pointers To Remember:

✓ Tighten abs and waist as you twist from side to side
✓ Twist torso with head and eyes following arm movement
✓ Maintain slight bend in knees throughout move
✓ Keep your back straight during motion
✓ Keep hips and feet facing forward
✓ Move slowly and under control

Common Mistakes To Avoid:

✓ Locking knees throughout motion
✓ Swinging object to gain momentum
✓ Rotating too far
✓ Jerking head
✓ Leaning forward/bending from the waist
✓ Looking down
✓ Moving too quickly

VARIATIONS

Beginners:

✓ Use only body weight—hands only with no object
✓ Keep object (water bottle) close to body
✓ Decrease range of motion—twist only slightly from side to side
✓ Perform movement seated in a chair
✓ Perform less repetitions

Intermediate/Advanced:

✓ Raise weighted object higher (e.g. chest level)
✓ Use two weighted objects: one for each hand
✓ Raise arms out to the side at shoulder level
✓ Use heavier object(s): (dumbbell, kettle bell, medicine ball, barbell, exercise machine)
✓ Rotate your back foot for greater range of motion
✓ Move explosively throughout motion

FAQ

How can I get the most out of my Twist Moves? Perform the Twist Moves throughout your work day. See page 123 for ideas on how to incorporate them into your day.

How often should I perform Twist Moves? If you are performing low-repetition twist movements with light resistance or no resistance, you can perform the moves daily. But, if you are performing twist strengthening exercises with added weights or resistance, it is recommended to perform them every other day, or two to three days per week. It is recommended that you give your body 24–48 hours to properly recover after a challenging twist workout. You can perform the Simple Twist Moves (shared on the previous page) at work in the office or break-room, or at home.

NOTE: You can progress from beginner to more challenging levels as you improve. See instructions for the Simple Twist Moves on page 124. Also, be sure and assess your twist to see how you are doing and how much you improve. **It is recommended that you perform the Twist Test on page 126 every four to six weeks to see how you are improving.**

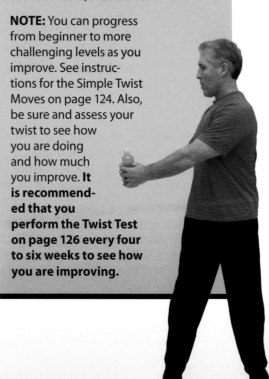

It's time to test your…
Twist

Now, try this test…

Twist Test #1: Standing Twist

Having a flexible and mobile upper and lower back is crucial to helping you throughout your busy work day, as well as preventing injury. To test the flexibility of your torso, let me introduce you to the Twist Test. This test measures the mobility and flexibility of your upper and lower back, shoulders and core muscles (waist, abs, and hips).

➤ GET READY

You'll need a non-slip surface to stand on, ruler or tape measure, chalk or colored masking tape (electrical or painters tape works well) and a wall, as well as a partner to assist in scoring your results. Place a 20-inch vertical line on a smooth wall.

➤ GET SET

Stand approximately an arm's distance from the wall with your body centered along the vertical line, keeping your back to the wall, feet shoulder-width apart and knees slightly bent.

➤ GO

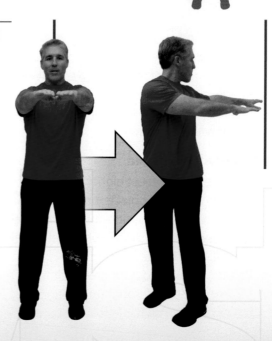

1. Next, extend your hands and arms in front of you and raise them to shoulder level, making them parallel to the floor.

2. Begin the test by slowly twisting your torso, and while reaching your hands and arms behind you as far as you safely and comfortably can, try to touch the wall with your fingertips. Remember to keep your feet facing forward throughout the test.

3. Have a friend, colleague or family member mark where the fingertips of your right hand touch the wall. Measure the distance from your fingertip mark to the vertical line. If you went past the line, score a positive result. If you did not go past the line, score your results in the negative.

4. Repeat steps 1-3, but this time to the left. Now add your scores together and divide by 2 to get your average. Perform the test one to two times on each side and take your best score.

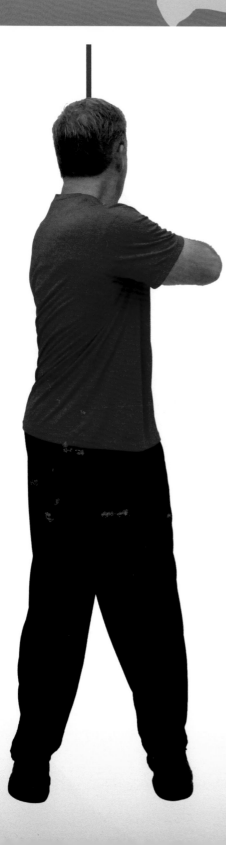

FINISH

The test is completed when:

✓ You have touched the wall and measured distance from the line
✓ You cannot touch the wall
✓ You use momentum to propel your body further
✓ You turn your feet to the side
✓ You experience discomfort or pain in your neck, lower back or knees

YOUR SCORE

See how you did by comparing your score with the scores below. Circle how you scored.

RATING	SCORE
Excellent	8 inches (20 centimeters)
Very Good	6 inches (15 centimeters)
Good	4 inches (10 centimeters)
Average	2 inches (5 centimeters)
Poor	0 inches (0 centimeters)

NOTE: It is important when performing this twisting test not to rotate beyond your ability or move too quickly, as this may cause discomfort in your upper or lower back or knees. Also, if you have back or knee problems it is recommended that you not perform this test.

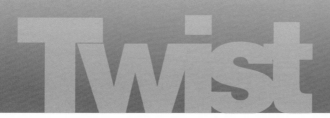

Twist Programs, Tools And Personality Profile Recommendations

To improve your twist, you can perform simple movements like those mentioned on pages 124–125, or, select twist activities from this chart containing various recommended programs and tools based upon your Fitness That Works Personality Profile. Note: All programs, tools or activities that are checked are recommended for you.

Fitness Personality Profile—My Personality Profile Is

▼   Check three that are the most appealing to you.

PUSH-PULL ACTIVITIES/EXERCISES	PROFILE A	PROFILE B	PROFILE C
☐ Simple Moves - Twist (With Water Bottle) (See pages 124–125)	✓	✓	✓
☐ Free Weights: Dumbbells and/or Barbells	✓		
☐ Medicine Ball	✓		
☐ Resistance Tubing	✓		
☐ Stability Ball	✓		
☐ Cables	✓		
☐ Kettle Bells	✓		
☐ Wood Chopping	✓		✓
☐ Strength Resistance Machines (e.g. Captains Chair, Cybex, or Life Fitness)	✓		
☐ Suspension Training (e.g. TRX, FKPro or Aerosling)	✓	✓	
☐ Sand Bags	✓		
☐ Fitness Classes (e.g. Pilates, Jazzercise, Zumba, Circuit Classes)		✓	✓
☐ Strength Training DVDs (e.g. 4321 Fitness, Insanity, P-90X, Body Blast)	✓		
☐ Martial Arts (e.g. Karate, Judo, Chun Kuk Do, Jeet Kune Do, Taekwondo)	✓		
☐ Golf		✓	✓
☐ Softball/Baseball		✓	✓
☐ Discus or Hammer Throwing		✓	✓
☐ Diving		✓	✓
☐ Hockey (In-Line and Ice)		✓	✓
☐ Racquet Sports (e.g. Tennis, Racquetball, Badminton, Lacrosse, Polo, Ping Pong)		✓	✓
☐ Dance (e.g. Hip-Hop, Ballet, Belly Dance)		✓	
☐ Wrestling (Sumo, Free Style, Greco)		✓	✓
☐ 4-3-2-1 Fitness Training (See pages 148–149)	✓	✓	✓

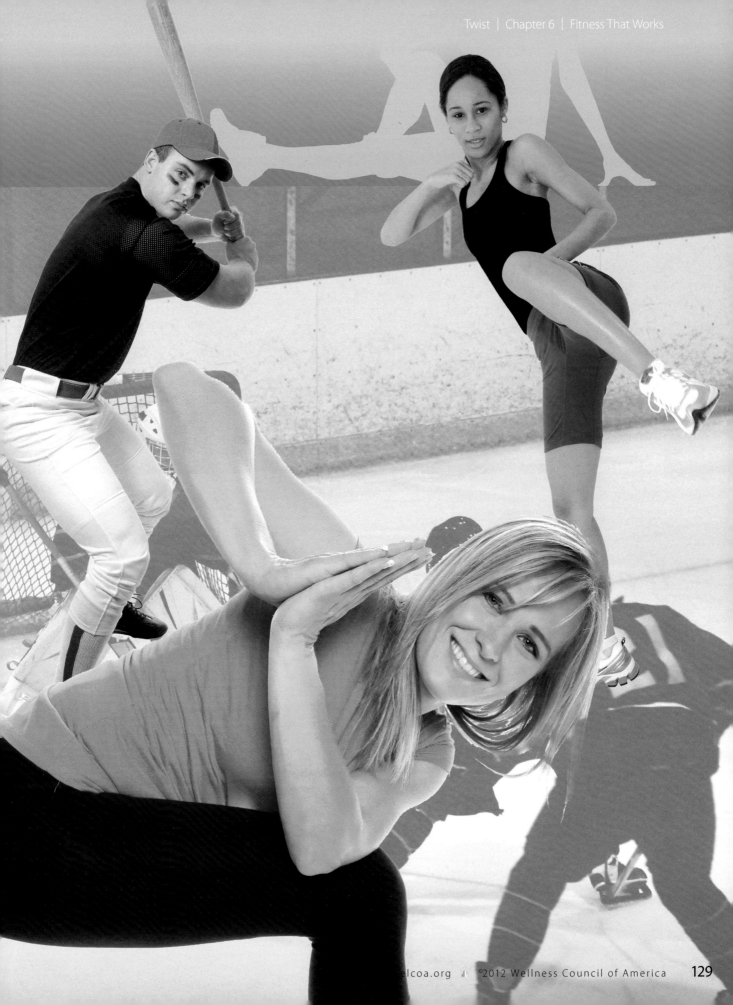

Lunge

"If everyone is moving forward together, then success takes care of itself.

—Henry Ford

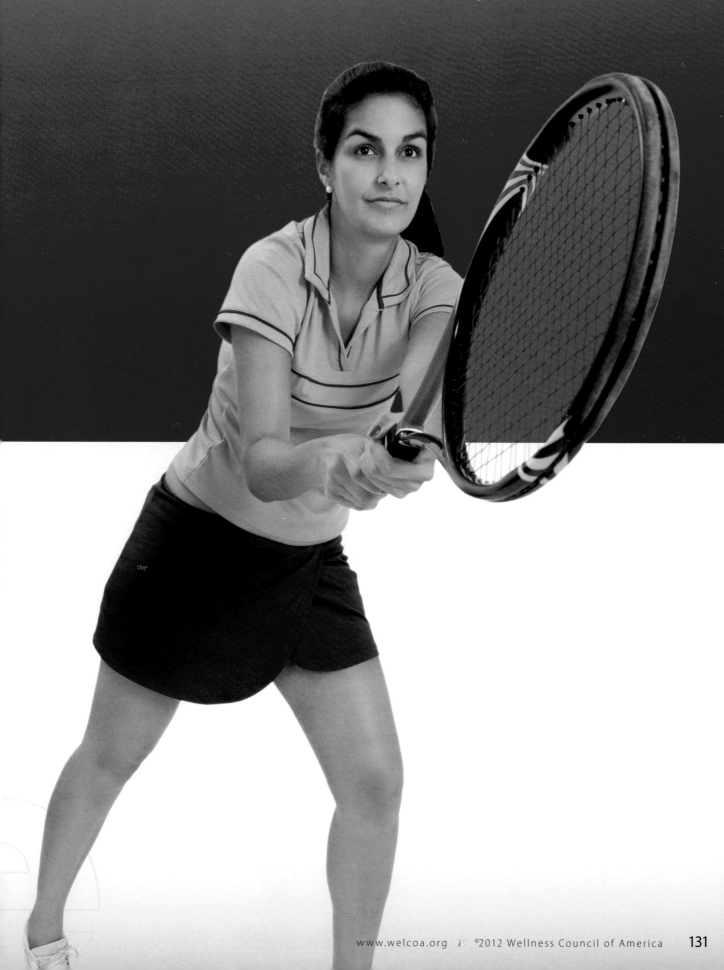

Lunge

AFTER READING THROUGH THE LAST SIX CHAPTERS OF THIS BOOK, I HOPE YOU'VE BEEN ENCOURAGED TO "MOVE" FORWARD.

Even if you've only moved a little bit, you are moving in the right direction. As we have discovered thus far with *Fitness That Works*, even the simplest of moves performed at work (or home) creates momentum and success that "takes care of itself." Why? Simple Moves make us feel better and moving for fitness eventually becomes a habit we begin to crave. In this chapter, I want to keep you moving and add to your success by introducing you to our last and final Simple Move: "lunge," and show you how easy it is to make it work at work.

We will explore:

1   What is lunge?

2   Why is lunge so important?

3   How to ensure your success

4   Simple moves you can do to improve your lunge

5   How to test your lunge

6   Recommended lunge programs, tools and much more

All For One And One For All!

While working in corporate health and fitness over the last 20 years, I have had the unique opportunity to see what works and what doesn't when it comes to motivating people to move. As you have seen throughout this book, performing the Simple Moves throughout your day really works. Along with Simple Moves, I want to share another tool that I have found can dramatically impact your future fitness success: ***teamwork!***

Research demonstrates that being a part of a group of like-minded individuals striving towards a common goal can profoundly impact success. I remember first learning this reality when we did the pilot testing of the Simple Moves with a group of 141 employees at a manufacturing facility in Orange County, California. At first, the management was a little reluctant, but as we shared the potential impact that teamwork could have on morale, corporate culture, productivity and a host of other benefits, they quickly got on board. In fact, they began to enlist employees as "ambassadors and trainers" to help

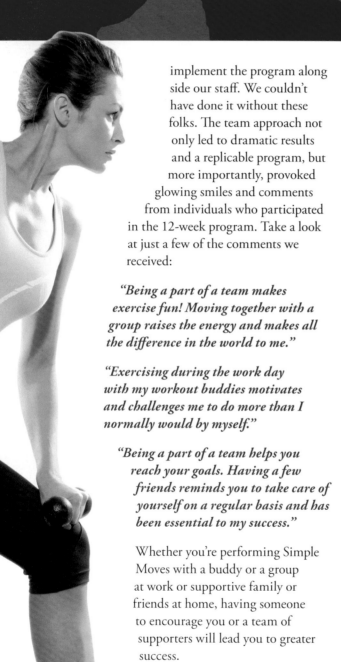

implement the program along side our staff. We couldn't have done it without these folks. The team approach not only led to dramatic results and a replicable program, but more importantly, provoked glowing smiles and comments from individuals who participated in the 12-week program. Take a look at just a few of the comments we received:

"Being a part of a team makes exercise fun! Moving together with a group raises the energy and makes all the difference in the world to me."

"Exercising during the work day with my workout buddies motivates and challenges me to do more than I normally would by myself."

"Being a part of a team helps you reach your goals. Having a few friends reminds you to take care of yourself on a regular basis and has been essential to my success."

Whether you're performing Simple Moves with a buddy or a group at work or supportive family or friends at home, having someone to encourage you or a team of supporters will lead you to greater success.

What Is Lunge?

When you hear the word "lunge," you may immediately think of a fencer with a sword, lunging to attack an opponent. If that's the picture in your head, you are not far off. The dictionary defines "lunge" as: "a quick thrust or jab usually made by leaning or striding forward."

The motion of lunge is something we all do every day. For example, we lunge when we bend down to tie our shoes, or pick up the morning paper or when opening a low filing cabinet or stepping over a pile of books on the floor. The motion of lunge is also one of the most common motions in sports and recreational activities.

Whether you are playing sports or moving throughout your day, all of these lunge activities require the entire lower body (thigh, buttocks, hamstrings, calf) and core (abs, hips and back) to work in coordination with one another.

How To Improve Your Lunge

Since the lunge motion is primarily a resistance training motion that we've previously discussed (see Push-Pull, Chapter 4), you can review the benefits of these two types of strength training again on pages 86–87.

How To Guarantee Your Success: How would you like to dramatically increase your ability to succeed in moving your body on a regular basis? All you need is a little teamwork. MIT research published in the *Journal of Science* in December 2011 studied the power of teamwork by analyzing the support of online social networking and the concept of "health buddies." The study demonstrated that individuals were three times more likely to adopt healthy behaviors (such as exercising more and eating healthy) if they were matched with others who had similar characteristics and interests. This is evidence that group support, even if you find it online, can be a powerful tool in your *Fitness That Works* toolbox!

Lunge

Here are four tips to help you ensure your
Fitness That Works **success:**

1 **Get a Buddy:** Think about enlisting the support of a colleague at work or family member or friend at home who has similar interests to you. Share with them your desire to start moving more and ask them if they would be ok with checking in on you (on a daily, weekly or bi-weekly basis). Chances are they will ask you if they can join in with you.

2 **Form a Team:** You can also put the power of more people to work for you by starting or joining a *Fitness That Works/Simple Moves* fitness group or team. You'll just need a group of like-minded individuals who are willing to use the concepts in this book and commit to moving their bodies along with you.

Here are some ways to connect with your team:

- Email or use Facebook or Twitter to plan your day before it begins: "I'm going to do a Simple Move every hour today…how about you?"
- Text one another periodically throughout the day by reporting: "I took the stairs before work today…how about you?"
- Invite coworkers to meet you in a location at your work to do your Simple Moves together: "Let's do some lunges in the break room after lunch, ok?"

Your Simple Moves team will share not only enthusiasm and encouragement with each other, but also tips for success and tried-and-true advice that will make your journey easier.

3 **Issue a Challenge:** Consider launching a four, eight or 12-week "Fitness That Works Challenge!" Challenge individuals from your department, work shift or anyone in your company to compete in a Simple Moves Challenge with the goal of seeing who can move the most throughout their workday over a designated period of time. It can be an individual challenge or a team approach. You can award winners who move the most with various prizes, as well as motivate one another with friendly competition throughout the duration of the program.

4 **Train others:** One of the best strategies to help get yourself moving is by helping someone else. Consider taking the concepts and moves found in this book and other Simple Moves workouts, and offer your support to others. Not only will you help those you care about, but you'll also be helping yourself to stick with your own Simple Moves program.

For more information on *Fitness That Works* Trainings, Webinars and onsite seminars go to: **www.pwsolutions.co**.

WHO'S ON YOUR TEAM

As you begin to think about applying all you've learned from this book and start moving your body more at work, take a moment to answer the following questions below. These are designed to help you develop your support team.

- How would you rate your current level of support? (Please circle one response below).

    Low (I'm really in need of some encouragement and accountability).

    Moderate (I have adequate support right now).

    High (I have all the support I need to be healthy and fit).

- Think of your friends/colleagues at work. Make a list of your top five "support team" members who could provide encouragement to you and who may benefit from a program like this.

> " *The strength of the team is each individual member... the strength of each member is the team.* "

— **Phil Jackson**
Future Basketball
Hall of Fame Coach

Lunge Moves & Lunge Tests That Work At Work
Try the moves and tests on the following pages to help improve your lunge!

It's time to improve your…
Lunge

Now, try this move…

Lunge Move #1: Elevated Lunge

Our last and final move of the book, lunge, is one of the best ways to help you reach your health and fitness goals. Let's take a look at a how you can improve your lunge.

➤ GET READY

This simple move is a very effective way to strengthen your entire lower body even from 9 to 5 while you're at work. Picture yourself, every hour or so, standing up from your desk or work station and performing this Simple Move. All you'll need is a non-slip surface to stand on, a non-moving chair, bench or stable object to place your foot on, and if you'd like, some form of added resistance (such as a pair of water bottles).

➤ GET SET

Stand approximately three feet away from a chair (with your back to the chair). Next, place your left foot on top of the chair while standing in a lunge or "split squat" position (right knee slightly bent) with hands and arms by your sides.

➤ GO

1. Begin the exercise by bending your right knee and lowering your center of gravity and left knee down towards the ground as far as you comfortably can and hold.

2. Pressing from the heel of the right (front) foot, straighten your leg and extend your hip to the standing step 1 position.

3. Repeat steps 1-2, eight to 20 times or as many as you can safely complete, then switch sides and repeat on the other leg.

NOTE: If you have knee problems, it is recommended that you either modify this move or select a different lower body exercise.

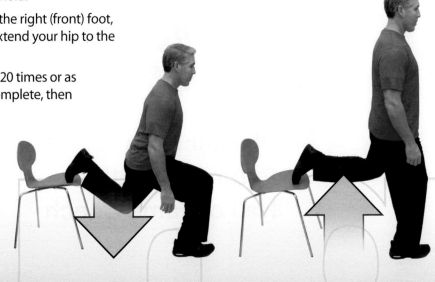

MAINTAIN PROPER FORM

Pointers To Remember:

✓ Keep body tall and straight
✓ Chin should be parallel to the floor
✓ Go down as low as you comfortably can
✓ Front knee should be slightly bent in standing position
✓ Front knee should be midline of your front foot
✓ Move slowly and under control

Common Mistakes To Avoid:

✓ Bending from the waist
✓ Looking down
✓ Locking front knee
✓ Going down too low
✓ Extending knee past front foot
✓ Moving too quickly

VARIATIONS

Beginners:

✓ Use only body weight
✓ Place arms in front of you for counter balance
✓ Decrease range of motion—lower body down ¼
✓ Hold lunge position without moving for 30-60 seconds
✓ Perform movement without elevating foot
✓ Perform less repetitions

Intermediate/Advanced:

✓ Use weights or added resistance (Water bottles, Dumbbell, Medicine ball)
✓ Increase range of motion (go lower)
✓ Descend slower
✓ Increase repetitions

FAQ

How can I get the most out of my Lunge Moves? Perform the lunge moves throughout your workday. Refer to Lunge Move #1: Elevated Lunge on the previous page for ideas on how to incorporate this move into your day.

How often should I perform my Lunge Moves? If you are performing low-repetition lunge movements with no resistance, you can perform the moves daily. But, if you are performing lunge strengthening exercises with added weights or resistance, it is recommended to give your body 24-48 hours to properly recover after a challenging lunge workout.

You can perform the Simple Lunge Moves shared on the previous page at work (in the office or break-room), or at home. **Note:** Depending upon your personality, see what works best for you on page 140.

NOTE: You can progress from beginner to more challenging levels as you improve. See instructions for the Simple Lunge Moves on the previous page. Also, be sure and test your lunge to see how you are doing and how much you improve.

NOTE: It is recommended that you perform the Lunge Test on page 138 every four to six weeks to see how you are improving.

It's time to test your…
Lunge

Now, try this test…

Lunge Test #1: Single Leg Lunge Test

Now that you've practiced your Lunge Moves That Work, let's take a moment to assess your lower body endurance and strength.

➤ GET READY

You'll need a non-slip surface to stand on, watch or timing device and optional chair for balance/support.

➤ GET SET

Stand with your hands and arms by your sides and your feet close together. Next, balance on your right foot by bending your left knee (approximately 60-90 degrees) and raising your left foot off the ground behind you).

➤ GO

1. Begin the test by lowering your center of gravity down, bending your right knee and lunging as if you were sitting back in an imaginary chair with the goal of going as low as you can and touching your left foot to the ground (without straightening the left leg).

2. Once your left foot taps the floor extend your right leg and straighten your hips to the standing position of step 1.

3. Repeat steps 1-2, as many times as you can for 30 seconds and record how many times your foot touches the floor as your score. If your foot does not touch the ground, do not count the repetition. After recording, perform the Single Leg Lunge Test on the other leg.

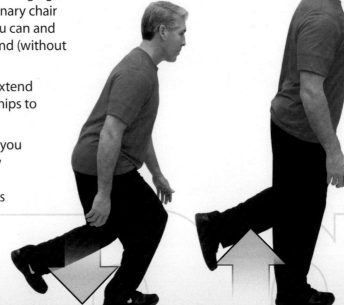

FINISH

The test is completed when:

✓ 30 seconds has elapsed
✓ You straighten your non-standing leg
✓ You experience discomfort or pain in your knees, hips or back

YOUR SCORE

See how you did by comparing your score with the scores below. Circle how you scored.

RATING	SCORE
Excellent	25+
Good	20-24
Average	11-19
Poor	11-19

" After recording, perform the Single Leg Lunge Test on the other leg. "

Lunge

Lunge Programs, Tools And Personality Profile Recommendations

To improve your lunge, you can perform simple movements like those mentioned on pages 136–137, or select lunge activities from this chart containing various recommended programs and tools based upon your Fitness That Works Personality Profile. Note: All programs, tools or activities that are checked are recommended for you.

Fitness Personality Profile—My Personality Profile Is

▼ Check three that are the most appealing to you.

LUNGE ACTIVITIES/EXERCISES	PROFILE A	PROFILE B	PROFILE C
☐ Simple Moves - One-Legged Elevated Lunge (See pages 136–137)	✓	✓	✓
☐ Free Weights: Dumbbells and/or Barbells	✓		
☐ Medicine Ball	✓		
☐ Resistance Tubing	✓		
☐ Stability Ball	✓		
☐ BOSU and/or Air Discs	✓		
☐ Kettle Bells	✓		
☐ Strength Cable Machines	✓		
☐ Suspension Training (e.g. TRX, FKPro or Aerosling)	✓	✓	
☐ Strength Fitness Classes (e.g. Circuit Classes, Boot Camps, etc.)		✓	✓
☐ Strength Training DVDs (e.g. Such as 4321 Fitness, Insanity, P-90X)	✓		
☐ Martial Arts (e.g. Karate, Judo, Chun Kuk Do, Jeet Kune Do, Taekwondo)	✓	✓	
☐ Fencing		✓	✓
☐ Sports (Football, Rugby, Baseball, Basketball, Softball, Soccer, Volleyball)		✓	✓
☐ Racquet Sports (e.g. Tennis, Racquetball, Badminton, Lacrosse, Polo, Ping Pong)		✓	✓
☐ Dance (e.g. Russian, Modern Jazz, Hip-Hop, Ballet)		✓	
☐ Wrestling (Free Style, Greco)		✓	✓
☐ 4–3–2–1 Fitness Training (See pages 148–149)	✓	✓	✓

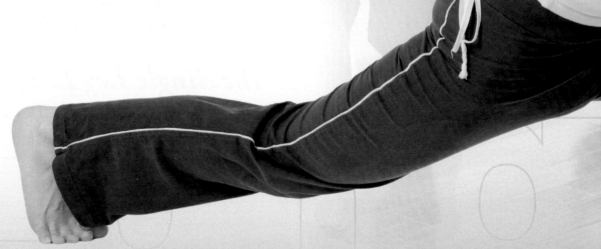

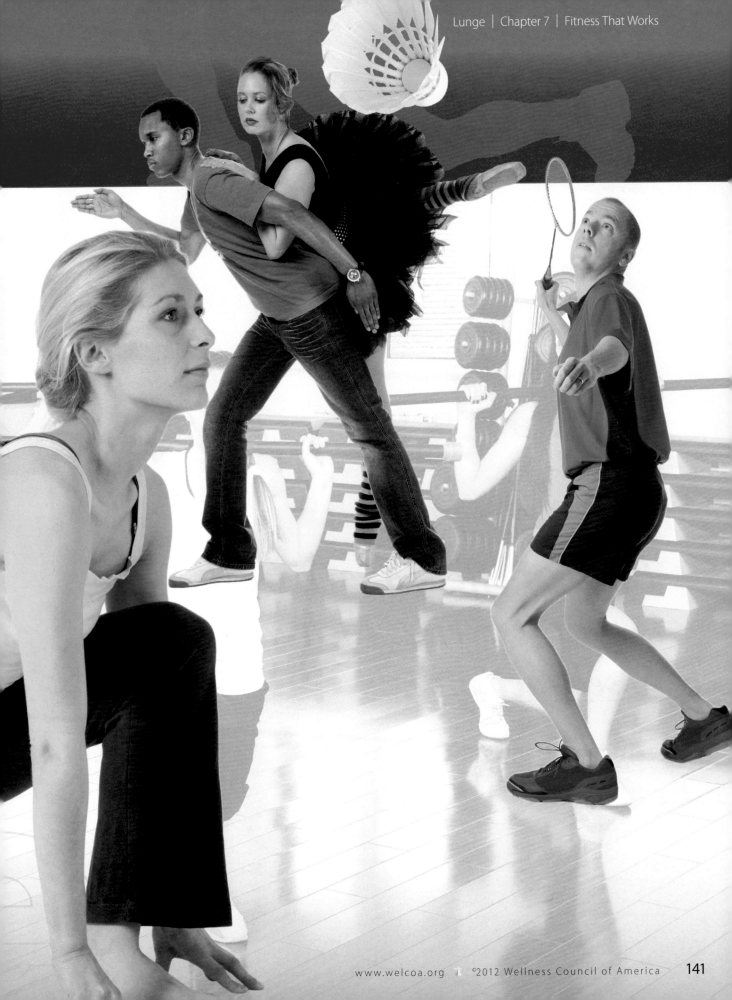

Make Your Move

"The best effect of any book is that it excites the reader to <u>self-activity</u>."

—Thomas Carlyle

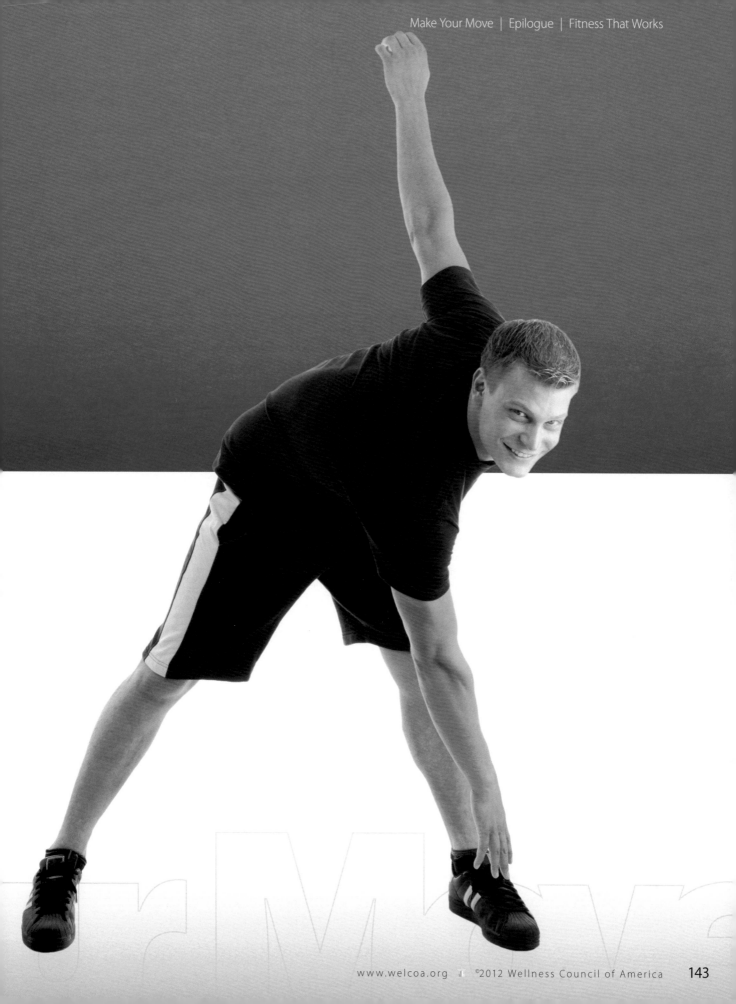

Now take just 10 steps to…

Make Your Move

Are You Ready To Make Your Move?

By completing the following steps in this chapter, you can design your own personal *Fitness That Works* plan and get moving.

1 **What do you want?** Take a moment to identify your goals. Write down your top one-to-three personal health areas you would most like to improve. (See pages 6–19).

1	2	3

2 **What makes you move?** Take a moment to identify what moves you most enjoy. Write down your top three activities. (See Introduction and Chapter 2, pages 6–19 and page 36–59).

1	2	3

3 **Take your first step.** List what potential personal benefits as well as any challenges you'd experience 4 or 12 weeks from today if you were to begin to "move" regularly. (See Chapter 3, pages 60–77).

4 **What's your "one thing?"** Ask yourself this question: "What's 'one thing' I'm not doing now that I can do (at work), and that if I did it on a regular basis, I know it would make a significant difference to my health and fitness?" Write your response below: (See Chapter 4, pages 78–99).

5 **Identify how much you sit.** For the next two days write down how much you sit at work and while commuting. (See Chapter 5, pages 100–115).

DAY 1 WORK	DAY 1 COMMUTE	DAY 2 WORK	DAY 2 COMMUTE

6 **What brings you joy?** List your top five "joy-filled" activities, games, sports or hobbies. (See Chapter 6, pages 116–129).

7 **Who's on your team?** Think of your friends and colleagues at work and make a list of your top five "support team" members. (See Chapter 7, pages 130–141).

8 **What's your next Move?** Determine what, when and how you are going to "move" and track your progress at work. You can select from this list, or create your own:

Fitness That Works—Simple Moves™:

☐ Simple One: 30:30™ (Perform one or more moves (shown below) for 30 seconds each, every 30 minutes at work).

☐ Simple 7™ (Perform all seven Moves from this book throughout your day).

☐ 4-3-2-1 Fitness™—10 Minute Total Body Breakthrough (See page 148–149 for more information).

☐ Other _____

Fitness That Works—Simple Moves™ Weekly Tracking Form

Using the weekly tracking form below, first, go to **MY SIMPLE MOVES** to review each move by referring to each indicated chapter and the page it is found on. Second, notate your ideas under **RELATED ACTIVITIES** by referring to the activities you wrote down in your Fitness Personality Profile—e.g. walking, basketball, Pilates. Third, under **COMPLETED MOVES**, check off the day and write down the time you did your moves. And last, under **MY POINTS**, award yourself one point per Simple Move completed, or three points for every 10 minutes of a related activity that you complete.

MY SIMPLE MOVES	RELATED ACTIVITIES	COMPLETED MOVES		MY POINTS
BALANCE (Ch. 1, Pg. 26) ➤ Standing One-Leg ➤ Walk The Line	_____ _____ _____ _____ _____	DAY: ☐ MON ☐ TUE ☐ WED ☐ THU ☐ FRI ☐ SAT ☐ SUN	TIME: _____ _____ _____ _____ _____ _____ _____	_____ _____ _____ _____ _____ _____ _____
REACH (Ch. 2, Pg. 48) ➤ Alternating Toe Touch ➤ Shoulder-Arm Circle	_____ _____ _____ _____ _____	DAY: ☐ MON ☐ TUE ☐ WED ☐ THU ☐ FRI ☐ SAT ☐ SUN	TIME: _____ _____ _____ _____ _____ _____ _____	_____ _____ _____ _____ _____ _____ _____
STEP (Ch. 3, Pg. 72) ➤ Stair-Stepping	_____ _____ _____ _____ _____	DAY: ☐ MON ☐ TUE ☐ WED ☐ THU ☐ FRI ☐ SAT ☐ SUN	TIME: _____ _____ _____ _____ _____ _____ _____	_____ _____ _____ _____ _____ _____ _____

(Continued on next page.)

Make Your Move

(Continued from previous page.)

Fitness That Works—Simple Moves™ Weekly Tracking Form *(Continued)*

MY SIMPLE MOVES	RELATED ACTIVITIES	COMPLETED MOVES		MY POINTS
PUSH-PULL (Ch. 4, Pg. 90) ➤ Chair Dip ➤ Shoulder Retraction Row		**DAY:** ☐ MON ☐ TUE ☐ WED ☐ THU ☐ FRI ☐ SAT ☐ SUN	**TIME:**	
SQUAT-LIFT (Ch. 5, Pg. 110) ➤ Squat-Lift		**DAY:** ☐ MON ☐ TUE ☐ WED ☐ THU ☐ FRI ☐ SAT ☐ SUN	**TIME:**	
TWIST (Ch. 6, Pg. 124) ➤ Standing Twist		**DAY:** ☐ MON ☐ TUE ☐ WED ☐ THU ☐ FRI ☐ SAT ☐ SUN	**TIME:**	
LUNGE (Ch. 7, Pg. 136) ➤ Elevated Lunge		**DAY:** ☐ MON ☐ TUE ☐ WED ☐ THU ☐ FRI ☐ SAT ☐ SUN	**TIME:**	

(Continued on next page.)

9 **What's your score?** Assess your fitness progress by recording how you score on the Simple Move tests in the chart below:

SIMPLE MOVE TEST	PAGE	DATE(S) TEST COMPLETED		SCORE	
Balance	30	#1	#2	#1	#2
Reach	52	#1	#2	#1	#2
Step	74	#1	#2	#1	#2
Push-Pull	94	#1	#2	#1	#2
Squat-Lift	112	#1	#2	#1	#2
Twist	126	#1	#2	#1	#2
Lunge	138	#1	#2	#1	#2

10 **Make A Movement!** Join us in challenging others to move more! If you're interested in motivating others in your company to move then check out our "Fitness That Works" seminars and educational resources by visiting our web site at www.pwsolutions.co. For more resources, try "Fitness @ the Speed of Life" at: www.4321fitness.com.

If you'd like daily contact, follow me on Twitter at coachseanfoy.

Here's wishing you "Fitness That Works!"

All the best today and always!

—Sean Foy, MA

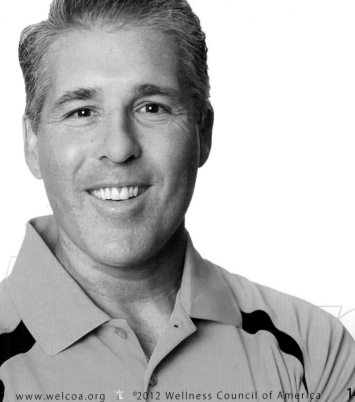

Also available from Sean Foy

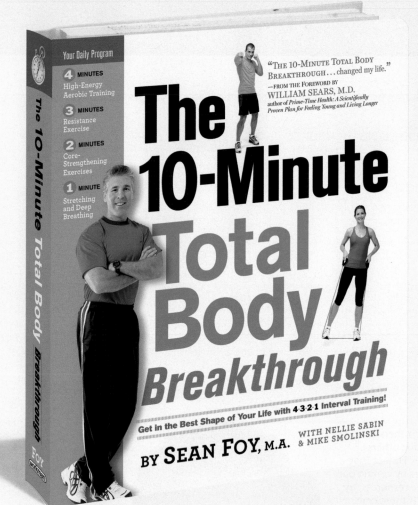

Includes quick-reference flip-cards to create hundreds of different workouts!

THE 10-MINUTE TOTAL BODY BREAKTHROUGH
by Sean Foy, M.A.

ISBN: 978-0-7611-5419-8
$22.95(US) $29.95(CAN)

Available wherever books are sold.

HR and Wellness professionals
Please contact specialmarkets@workman.com for special discounts on orders of 10 or more copies.

(workman)

www.workman.com | www.4321fitness.com

PRAISE FOR
4-3-2-1 Interval Training

"I really didn't see how working out for 10 minutes a day would make a difference, but it did! I went from 234 pounds to 200 in 12 weeks!"

–Denice Kennedy, grandmother of three

"By far the easiest and most user-friendly program I have ever found. I started to see results during the second week . . . I would recommend this program to anyone."

–Bill Hawkins, successful business owner

"Sean's program is extremely effective! I worked out for years on my own doing 10, 45, even 60 minutes' worth of cardio and not seeing results. I am working out less, but getting more results."

–Cathy Romero, mother of triplets and former aerobics instructor

How Does It Work?

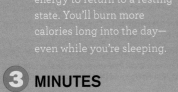

4 MINUTES
High-Energy Aerobic Training

Raising and then lowering intensity boosts metabolism, because your body uses energy to return to a resting state. You'll burn more calories long into the day—even while you're sleeping.

3 MINUTES
Resistance Exercise

Activating large muscle groups recruits significant energy from the smaller assisting muscles, which increases the overall calories you expend during the workout.

2 MINUTES
Core Training

Toning your midsection improves posture and strengthens lower back, hips, and abdomen—the key to avoiding back pain.

1 MINUTE
Stretching and Deep Breathing

Deep breathing calms the nervous system. It can reduce blood pressure levels and trigger the release of endorphins.

No Time? No Problem!

10 Minutes a Day Can Change Your Life!

Easy, fat-melting mini-workouts you can do anytime, anywhere—at your desk, in your hotel room, or at home in front of your TV!

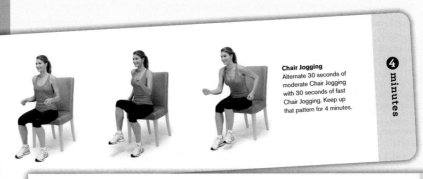

Chair Jogging
Alternate 30 seconds of moderate Chair Jogging with 30 seconds of fast Chair Jogging. Keep up that pattern for 4 minutes.

4 minutes

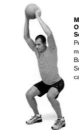
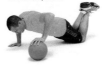
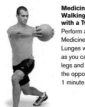

Medicine Ball Overhead Squat
Perform as many Medicine Ball Overhead Squats as you can in 1 minute.

Medicine Ball Knee Push-Up
Perform as many Medicine Ball Knee Push-Ups as you can in 1 minute, 30 seconds per arm.

Medicine Ball Walking Lunge with a Twist
Perform as many Medicine Ball Walking Lunges with a Twist as you can, alternating legs and twisting to the opposite side, in 1 minute.

3 minutes

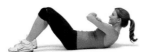
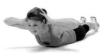

Crossed-Arms Ab Crunch
Perform as many Crossed-Arms Ab Crunches as you can in 1 minute.

Back Extension
Perform as many Back Extensions as you can (hold the upward position for 2 seconds and repeat) in 1 minute.

2 minutes

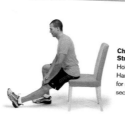
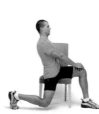

Chair Hamstring Stretch
Hold the Chair Hamstring Stretch for up to 15 seconds each leg.

Chair Thigh Stretch
Hold the Chair Thigh Stretch for up to 15 seconds each leg.

1 minute

RESOURCES AND REFERENCES

Introduction: Get Movin'
Athletic Body in Balance. Cook, Gray. (2003). Human Kinetics Publishing: Champaign.

Corrective exercise: "Move well and move often." From Gray Cook's Pearls of Wisdom, Part 2, FMS Course. (See: www.optimumsportsperformance.com)

The joint by joint approach. Gray Cook. (See: www.graycook.com)

Core Strength: A new model for injury prediction and prevention. Journal of Occupational Medicine and Toxicology, 2:3. (2007). doi:10.1186/1745-6673-2-3

Take 10: Simple Moves Research. Joe Leutzinger, PhD. (See: www.4321fitness.com)

Functional fitness: working out for real life functions. Shaw, G. (See: www.webmd.com)

Personality Quiz. American Institute for Cancer Research. Pamela Peeke, MD and Melanie Polk, RD. (See: "What's Your Workout Personality," www.webmd.com)

ADDITIONAL EXERCISE PERSONALITY TESTS:

The 8 Colors of Fitness. Brue, S. (April, 2008). Oakledge Press: Delray Beach.

What's your exercise personality? (See: www. sportsmedicine.about.com)

Just do it . . . before you talk yourself out of it: The self-talk of adults thinking about physical activity. Cousins, S.O. & Gillis, M.M. (2005). Psychology of Sport and Exercise, 6 (3), pp. 313–34.

Chapter 1: Balance
Athletic Body in Balance. Cook, Gray. (2003). Human Kinetics Publishing: Champaign.

Centers for Disease Control and Prevention/ National Center for Injury Prevention and Control (NCIPC). (See: www.cdc.gov, "Home and Recreational Safety")

Fall Proof: enhancing mobility and balance in older Americans. Rose, D. Titan Magazine. (See: www.titanmag.com/2005/fall_proof)

Prospective study of the impact of fear of falling on activities of daily living. Cumming. R.G., Salkeld, G., Thomas, M, et al. The Journals of Gerontology Series A Biological Science and Medical Science 55, pp. 299–305. (2000).

The science behind BOSU and balance training. (See: www.bosu.com)

Measuring Functional Fitness of Older Adults. Jones, C. J. & Rikl, E. The Journal on Active Aging. (March- April, 2002). (See: www.icaa.cc/1.../member.../ measuringfunctionalfitness2.pdf)

Interventions for Addressing Low Balance Confidence in Older Adults: A Systematic Review and Meta-Analysis. Rand, D., Carter, W.C., Yiu, J. & Eng, J. J. Age and Ageing, 40(3), pp. 297-306. (2011). Oxford University Press.

Stork Test. Practical Measurements For Evaluation In Physical Education, (4th Ed.). Johnson, B.L. & Nelson, J.K. (1979). Burgess: Minneapolis. (For other balance tests, see: www.topendsports.com)

Single Leg Balance Test to identify risk of ankle sprains. Trojian, T.H. & McKeag, D.B. British Journal of Sports Medicine, 40, pp. 610-613. (2006).

Standardized Field Sobriety Test: "Walk and Turn" Test. U.S. Department of Transportation, National Highway Traffic Safety Administration. (See: www.nhtsa.gov)

For additional Balance fitness tools and resources, see: www.4321fitness.com.

Chapter 2: Reach
Reach for the stars: "Sic Itur ad Astra:" Traditions Motto/Words. National Defense. (April 23, 2009). (See: www.rcaf-arc.forces.gc.ca)

Seniors and Exercise. American Academy of Orthopedic Surgeons. (February, 2008). (See www.orthoinfo.aaos.org, "Effects of Aging")

Ready to Roll. Michael Boyle. Training and Conditioning Magazine. (December, 2006).

Fascial Fitness: Training In The Neuromyofascial Web. (See: www.ideafit.com)

"Mobility vs. Flexibility: What's the difference?" (See: www.graycookmovement.com)

Flexibility training research. Dr. Len Kravitz. (See: www.drlenkravitz.com/Articles/flexibility.html)

Stretching Research Retrospective. Len Kravitz. Idea Fitness Journal. (2009). (See: www.ideafit.com/fitness-library)

Science of Flexibility, (2nd Ed.). Alter, M. J. (1996). Human Kinetics Publishing: Champaign, IL.

Measuring Functional Fitness of Older Adults. Jones, C.J. & Rikl, R.E. The Journal on Active Aging. (March-April, 2002). (See: www.icaa.cc/1.../member.../measuringfunctionalfitness2.pdf)

American College of Sports Medicine. ACSM's Guidelines for Exercise Testing and Prescription, 7th Edition. (2006). Lippincott Williams and Wilkins: Philadelphia.

Shoulder Flexibility Test. (See: www.sportsmedicine.about.com)

Movement. Cook, Gray (2011). On Target Publications: Santa Cruz.

National Institute on Aging. (See www.nia.nih.gov)

For additional Reach fitness tools and resources, see: www.4321fitness.com.

Chapter 3: Step
Aerobic Exercise. (See: www.medicinenet.com)

Fresh Start. The Stanford Medical School Health and Fitness Program. Farquhar, J. W. (1996). Stanford Medical School.

The Heart Rate Story. Ceconi, C., Guardigli, G., Rizzo, P., Francolini, G. & Ferrari, R. The European Heart Rate Journal Supplements. (September 1, 2011). Oxford University Press.

Cardiovascular System Facts. (See: www.pbs.org and www.encyclopedia.com)

Physical Activity Guidelines for Americans. U.S. Department of Health and Human Services. (2008). (See: www.nhlbi.nih.gov)

Dr. Kenneth Cooper: "The Father of Aerobics." (See: www.cooperinstitute.org)

Association of Long-Distance Corridor Walk Performance with Mortality, Cardiovascular Disease, Mobility Limitation and Disability. (May 3, 2006). Newman, A., et al. JAMA, p. 2018-2026.

Step Test. Adapted from The Canadian Home Fitness test (Canadian Public health Assoc. Project) and the YMCA Step Test. Golding, L. A., Myers, C. R., Sinning, W. E., Y's Way to Physical Fitness, 3rd ed., (1989) Human Kinetics Publishing: Champaign.

American College of Sports Medicine. ACSM's Guidelines for Exercise Testing and Prescription, 7th Edition. (2006). Lippincott, Williams and Wilkins: Philadelphia.

Exercise and aging. Can you walk away from Father Time? Harvard Men's Health Watch. (December, 2005). (See: www.health.harvard.edu)

A 30-year follow-up of the Dallas bed rest and training study: effect of age on cardiovascular adaptation to exercise training. McGuire, D.K., Levine, B.D., Williamson, J.W., et al. Circulation, 104, pp. 1358-1366. (2001). (See: http://circ.ahajournals.org)

Essentials of Strength Training and Conditioning. Baechle, T. R., et al. (2000).

Aerobics and Fitness Association of America. (See: www.afaa.com)

For additional Step fitness tools and resources, see: www.4321fitness.com.

Chapter 4: Push-Pull
Electromyographic analysis of the triceps brachii muscle during a variety of triceps exercises. Boehler, B. in Clinical Exercise Physiology. (J. Porcari, Ed.). (December, 2011). (See also: www.acefitness.org/certifiednews/images/article/pdfs/ACETricepsStudy.pdf)

The New Rules of Lifting. Schuler, L. & Cosgrove, A. (2006.) Penguin Books: New York.

Men's Health Big Book of Exercises. Campbell, A. (2009). Rodale, Inc.: New York.

Changes in dynamic exercise performance following a sequence of preconditioning isometric muscle actions. Journal of Strength and Conditioning Research, 17(4), 678–685 2003. (2006.) See also: National Strength & Conditioning Association.

Corporate Syndrome. (See: www.backintoit.com)

The enduring measure of fitness: the simple push-up. (See: www.nytimes.com)

Biomarkers: The 10 Determinants of Aging You Can Control. Evans, W. & Rosenberg, I. (1991.) Simon & Schulster: New York.

Pull-up tests. Adapted from Essentials of Strength Training and Conditioning. Baechle, T.R., Earle, R.W. (2008).

How many pull-ups should I be able to do? (See: www.livestrong.com)

Strong Women, Strong Bones. Nelson, Miriam. (2000). Putnam Books: New York.

Resistance Training Guidelines. Adapted from *The American College of Sports Medicine Strength Training Guidelines*, 2009.

Progression Models in Resistance Training for Healthy Adults. Jacobs, I. Medicine & Science in Sports & Exercise, 41(3), pp. 687-708. (March, 2009).

For additional Push-Pull fitness tools and resources, see: www.4321fitness.com.

Chapter 5: Squat-Lift

Canadian Fitness and Lifestyle Research Institute. George Sheehan, MD. *The Research File.* (2000). Reference No. 00-01.

Knee biomechanics of the dynamic squat exercise. Escamilla, R.F. *Medicine & Science in Sports & Exercise*, 33(1), pp. 127-41. (January, 2001).

Effect of Functional Exercise Training on Functional Fitness Levels of Older Adults. *Gundersen Lutheran Medical Journal*, 5(1). (July, 2008).

12 Reasons why every adult should strength train. (See: www.wellness.ma/adult-fitness/strength-training-12-reasons.htm)

Safety of the Squat Exercise, Current Comment from The American College of Sports Medicine, pp. 1-3. (March, 2000).

Sedentary behaviors increase risk of cardiovascular disease mortality in men. Warren, T.Y., Barry, V., Hooker, S.P., Sui, X., Church, T.S., & Blair, S.N. *Medicine & Science in Sports & Exercise*, 42(5), pp. 879-85. (May, 2010).

"The Cool Chair." (See: www.lazyboy.com)

Why your desk job is slowly killing you. (See: www.msnbc.com)

Sedentary behavior, physical activity and a continuous metabolic syndrome risk score in adults. Wijndaele, K., Duvigneaud, N., Matton, L., et al. *European Journal of Clinical Nutrition*, 63, pp. 421–429. (2009).

Phys Ed: The men who stare at screens. (See: www.well.blogs.nytimes.com)

Refining the exercise prescription to maintain muscle power as we age. Tufts University. (See: www.tufts.edu)

Healthy worksites create healthy communities. (Quote from Barbara E. Ainsworth, ACSM). (See: www.health.gov/paguidelines/blog)

Non-Exercise Activity Thermogenesis (NEAT). Levine, J.A. Nutrition Reviews, 62, pp. S82–S97. (2004).

Move A Little Lose A Lot. Levine, James (2009). Crown Publishers: New York.

Squat-Lift norms and test. Measuring functional fitness of older adults, Jones C.J., Rikli R.E., *The Journal on Active Aging*, March April 2002, pp. 24–30.

30-s. Chair-Stand Test as a Measure of Lower Body Strength in Community-Residing Older Adults. Jones, C. J., Rikli, R. E., Beam, W. *Research Quarterly for Exercise and Sport*, 70 (2), 113-119. (1999). (See also: www.topendsports.com)

Just Stand (See: www.juststand.org)

For additional Squat-Lift fitness tools and resources, see: www.4321fitness.com.

Chapter 6: Twist

"The Twist." Chubby Checker. (See: www.elyrics.net)

2011 Champions Of Health And Fitness—America's Doctor: Regina Benjamin, MD. (See: www.fitnessmagazine.com)

Super Abs Resource Manual: Power of Excellence. Len Kravitz, Ph.D. University of New Mexico. (See: www.unm.edu/~lkravitz)

Making Exercise Fun: Ways To Get Moving When You'd Rather Not. University of Virginia Health System. (See: www.uvahealth.com/blog)

Make Fitness Fun. (See: www.parade.com/health)

Top 10 Tips For Making Fitness Fun. (See: www.fitafterthirty.com)

Make Fitness Fun For The Whole Family. (See: www.familyfitness.about.com)

Wired for Joy: The Revolutionary Method for Creating Happiness from Within. Mellin, Laurel. (2010). Hay House.

Twist norms and test. Adapted from Nieman, David. *Exercise Testing and Prescription, trunk rotation flexibility tests.* (2003). McGraw Hill Publishers. (See also: Trunk Rotation Tests at www.topendsports.com)

Movement. Cook, Gray (2011). On Target Publications: Santa Cruz.

For additional Twist fitness tools and resources, see: www.4321fitness.com.

Chapter 7: Lunge

Social Networks and Health. *MIT researcher finds that social networks influence health behaviors.* (See: www. web.mit.edu)

An experimental study of homophily in the adoption of health behavior. Centola, D. *Science*, 334(6060), pp. 1269-1272. I: 10.1126/science.1207055 (December 2, 2011).

"Dynamic Trendelenburg:" Single-Leg-Squat Test for Gluteus Medius Strength. Livengood, A.L., DiMattia, M.A. & Uhl, T.L. *Athletic Therapy Today*, 9(1), pp. 24-25. (2004). (See: www.mc.uky.edu/athletic_training/Publications_2008_2.html)

What are the validity of the single-leg-squat test and its relationship to hip-abduction strength? DiMattia MA, Livengood AL, Uhl TL, Mattacola CG, Malone TR. *Journal of Sport Rehabilitation.* 14:108-123. (2005) Human Kinetics Publishers, Champaign, IL.

Lunge norms and test. 30-s. Chair-Stand Test as a Measure of Lower Body Strength in Community-Residing Older Adults. Jones, C. J., Rikli, R. E., Beam, W. *Research Quarterly for Exercise and Sport,* 70 (2), 113-119. (1999) (See also: www. topendsports.com)

American Council on Exercise. (See: www.acefitness.org)

Division of Nutrition, Physical Activity and Obesity. (See: www.cdc.gov/nccdphp)

For additional Lunge fitness tools and resources, see: www.4321fitness.com.

Epilogue: Make Your Move

7 Habits of Highly Effective People. Covey, Stephen R. (1989). Free Press.

Fitness That Works-Simple Moves™. (See: www.pwsolutions.co)

Fitness @ The Speed of Life™. (See: www.4321fitness.com)

American Alliance for Health, Physical Education, Recreation and Dance. (See: www.aahperd.org)

Idea Health and Fitness Association (See: www.ideafit.com)

Let's Move: (See: www.letsmove.gov)

National Strength and Conditioning Association: (See: www.nsca-lift.org)

National Institute of Health (See: www.nih.gov)

Office of the Surgeon General (See: www.surgeongeneral.gov)

Special Olympics International: (See: www.specialolympics.org)

YMCA and YWCA: (See: www.ymca.net and www.ywca.org)

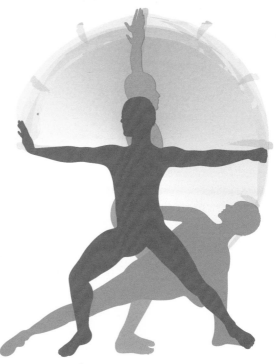